# BODIES IN FLUX

# BODIES IN FLUX

## SCIENTIFIC METHODS FOR

## NEGOTIATING MEDICAL UNCERTAINTY

## CHRISTA TESTON

THE UNIVERSITY OF CHICAGO PRESS

Chicago and London

The University of Chicago Press, Chicago 60637
The University of Chicago Press, Ltd., London
© 2017 by The University of Chicago

Published 2017

Printed in the United States of America

26 25 24 23 22 21 20 19 18 17   1 2 3 4 5

ISBN-13: 978-0-226-45052-0 (cloth)
ISBN-13: 978-0-226-45066-7 (paper)
ISBN-13: 978-0-226-45083-4 (e-book)
DOI: 10.7208/chicago/9780226450834/001.0001

Library of Congress Cataloging-in-Publication Data
Names: Teston, Christa, author.
Title: Bodies in flux : scientific methods for negotiating
medical uncertainty / Christa Teston.
Description: Chicago ; London : The University of Chicago Press, 2017. |
Includes bibliographical references and index.
Identifiers: LCCN 2016038464| ISBN 9780226450520 (cloth : alk. paper) |
ISBN 9780226450667 (pbk. : alk. paper) | ISBN 9780226450834 (e-book)
Subjects: LCSH: Evidence-based medicine. | Uncertainty (Information theory)
Classification: LCC R723.7 .T47 2017 | DDC 616—dc23
LC record available at https://lccn.loc.gov/2016038464

♾ This paper meets the requirements of
ANSI/NISO Z39.48–1992 (Permanence of Paper).

*For Lolly and Paw, with love*

# CONTENTS

# ACKNOWLEDGMENTS

The wise eyes and kind minds of countless colleagues, friends, and loved ones helped make this book what it is. We all have those people in our lives who help prepare us for the things we don't yet know we're going to write. For this, I offer thanks to Casey Boyle, Jim Brown, Davida Charney, William Hart-Davidson, Scott Graham, Brian McNely, Margaret Price, Nathaniel Rivers, Chad Wickman, and Greg Wilson. You may not have known it, but our back-stage brainstorming at conferences, seminars, and through various social media and e-mail exchanges helped shape this book.

So many of you gave of your time and suffered through early prose, under-developed drafts, and half-baked ideas. You are priceless. For their kindness, patience, and disciplinary expertise, I am grateful to Ellen Barton, Jonathan Buehl, Scott DeWitt, Wendy Hesford, Candice Lanius, Jim Phelan, Thomas Rickert, Cindy Selfe, Clay Spinuzzi, Pamela Takayoshi, Karen Thompson, and the three anonymous peer reviewers whose revision recommendations were worth their weight in gold.

Informal conversations and interviews with a host of experts in science and medicine also influenced how I conceive of doing rhetoric while dwelling in a world full of contingencies. For this, I am thankful to the kind folks in the Ohio State University's Division of Human Genetics, the College of Public Health, and departments of pathology, mathematics, psychology, and statistics. I'm thankful to the Association of Teachers of Technical Writing (http://www.attw.org) and *Technical Communication Quarterly* for allowing me to adapt for chapter 2 of this book portions of my (2012) article, "Moving from Artifact to Action: A Grounded Investigation of Visual Displays of Evidence during Medical Deliberations."

It is a privilege to work alongside budding scholars who are also interested in questions about how to make more livable worlds. I am especially grateful to the graduate students in my fall 2015 Research Methods Seminar who, without knowing it, were in so many ways this book's very first audience.

Other institutional structures and actors helped bring this book to fruition, including the graduate program at Kent State University from which I hail. Its founder, the late Stephen P. Witte, made the study of workplace writing and literacy in Kent State's Literacy, Rhetoric, and Social Practice program possible. And although I never met the man, I could swear he sat on my shoulder the entire time I drafted this book. Christina Haas taught me how to capture complexity—to be truly attuned to people, places, and things for the ways they affect human behavior and future action: thank you, "Dr. Haas." And to Raymond Craig, who taught me what it means to chop wood, carry water—I am appreciative. I'm also grateful for the early and crucial support of all of my former colleagues in the Department of Writing Arts at Rowan University and for my friends and former colleagues in the Department of English at University of Idaho. Thanks especially to Jodie Nicotra, Karen Thompson, and Gary Williams. And to my other Palouse partners in crime— Belle Baggs, Teressa Benz, Dylan Champagne, Casey Doyle, Stacy Isenbarger, Mario Montes, Caro Caro P, and Alexandra Teague—you saved my life.

Finally, there are those folks who make sure you eat and drink more than nut thins and Diet Coke while furiously writing, rewriting, and revising— the people who forgive your obsessive compulsion to make everything sound just right. Thank you Christopher Elliott for being my go-to guy. Thank you Molly Farrell for self-care pie. Thank you mom and dad for keeping me sane when things fall apart and the center cannot hold. Thank you Koda and Raja for your fuzzy and unfailing love. And seriously: thank you Columbus, Ohio, Jimmy John's bicycle delivery guys for your endless supply of speedily delivered number sixes.

*Acknowledgments*

# 1. EVIDENTIAL MATTER(S)

*Not only is everything changing, but all is flux.*
*That is to say, what is is the process of becoming itself,*
*while all objects, events, entities, conditions, structures, etc.,*
*are forms that can be abstracted from this process.*
David Bohm, *Wholeness and the Implicate Order*

*Medicine is a heterogeneous coalition of ways of handling bodies,*
*studying pictures, making numbers, conducting conversations....*
*There is multiplicity even inside medicine's biomedical "core."*
Annemarie Mol and Marc Berg,
introduction to *Differences in Medicine*

After gradual loss of his mobility and speech, on June 17, 2014, my paternal grandfather died of multiple system atrophy—a rare and relatively mysterious degenerative disease that affects the brain. Fewer than twelve months later, at only age fifty-nine, my uncle died of an aggressive form of brain cancer. As I grieve for my grandmother, Bernice, who in one year lost both her son-in-law and her life partner of five decades, I am struck by the degree to which medical professionals struggled to name and navigate our loved ones' illnesses. Because disease seemed to sneak up on my grandfather and uncle and then slowly whittle away at their brains and bodies, I've become hyper-aware of my father's tendency to repeat a story for the second or third time. When dad suffers a minor injury now and then because of what appears to be mere clumsiness or overexertion, I worry. Concerned that his forgetfulness, muscle pulls, and pain might be signs or symptoms of something ominous, I try and take comfort in recent medical tests and scans that indicate dad's brain and body are in pretty good shape.

Uncertainty posed by the ambiguous space between living and dying is mitigated, albeit only in part, through medical evidence. But how are evidential worlds assembled from bodies in perpetual flux? From where does medicine's evidential weight hail? What protocols and procedures elevate everyday biological activities to positions of argumentative authority? This book seeks answers to such questions through an exploration of the backstage, behind-the-scenes biomedical practices that materially render medical evidence both visible and actionable. *Bodies in Flux* is inspired by medical professionals' success with and failures at navigating not knowing. Each chapter investigates one of four specific scientific methods for negotiating medical uncertainty in cancer care: evidential visualization, evidential assessment, evidential synthesis, and evidential computation.

Defining and diagnosing disease is a kind of quixotic empiricism. It requires taking what's known now and making best guesses about what's to come. Yet, as physicist and philosopher David Bohm (1981) argues, "all is flux" (61). Inspired by partnerships with nature, premodern medical and scientific practitioners once used astrological evidence to manage bodily flux. For example, constellations once aided in predicting astral circumstances of birth, controlling parts of a body, and determining when and where to let blood or take medicine (French 2003, 132). Today's attempts at managing bodily flux involve monitoring corporeal symptoms and modeling risks. From telescopes to stethoscopes to microscopes, biomedical projections have always resulted from human and nonhuman partnerships. The always already collaborative nature of attempts at forecasting corporeal futures complicates contemporary biomedical practice and precision. *Bodies in Flux* explores such complications.

I invoke "flux" not only in reference to cancer care's corporeal contingencies but also to orient readers' attention toward scientific indeterminacy (Barad 2007)—the kind of contingencies and indeterminacy that Heraclitus may have had in mind when he famously declared the impossibility of stepping into the same river twice. As a concept, flux highlights the evidential complexity of being (a body) in the world. In rhetorical theory, flux counters the notion that rhetoric, and decision making in particular, consists of discrete and autonomous elements such as audience, purpose, or context. Contesting the reductive nature of *a* or *the* rhetorical situation, Jenny Edbauer (2005), Louise Weatherbee Phelps (1991), Laurie Gries (2015), and several other rhetoric scholars have advocated for an ecological view of rhetoric that situates suasive activity within (and because of) a "wider sphere of active, historical, and lived processes" (Edbauer 2005, 8). An ecological model of rhetoric characterizes "rhetoric" as a verb. A performance. A constant process of unpredictable unfolding. To study rhetoric, therefore, is to study flux and flow. To study rhetoric is to explore processes of becoming (Bohm 1981).

In the following chapters, I trace processes of becoming in the biomedical backstage. That is, I trace how modern medicine *does* rhetorical work. To do this, I identify and analyze biomedical practitioners' material-discursive negotiations with matter, movement, and time. I do so motivated by the troubling awareness that well prior to medical practitioners' attempts at understanding my grandfather's, uncle's, and father's corporeal conditions through freeze-framed abstractions (such as medical images or blood tests), processes

deep within their bodies were and are always at work. Material actions—
some seen, some unseen—perform our bodily being long before doctors even
know to look.

*Bodies in Flux* is about and for those who compose, communicate, contend, and cope with biomedical evidence as material made to mean. Each
chapter's investigation of medical practitioners' attempts at managing bodies'
inherent indeterminacy is written with patients, practitioners, policy makers,
technical communicators, rhetoricians, medical humanists, and science and
technology scholars in mind. Exigencies for a book about how biomedical evidence is made to mean are abundant. In response to evidence-based
medicine's fetishization of medical evidence many wonder: Whose evidence?
What counts as evidence? And how is evidence tallied and made to matter?
Commoditized, direct-to-consumer genetic testing kits and government-
mandated electronic medical records invite additional scrutiny: Who owns
my medical evidence? Who should or should not have access to it? Evidential
complexities such as these have implications not just for decision making.
Evidential complexities such as these also have economic and ethical effects.

The rate of women in the United States choosing to undergo what is now
referred to as a "bilateral risk-reducing mastectomy" has increased by 50 percent in just the last five years. As I write this, these rates, along with what is
colloquially referred to as the "Angelina Jolie effect," have sparked a cultural
firestorm of debate about medical certainty, women's choice, and biomedical
ethics. In an effort to demystify (if not normalize) the procedural and surgical implications of her decision to undergo a preventative double mastectomy, Jolie (2013) detailed three months of medical procedures and experiences in a *New York Times* op-ed. Since the op-ed's publication, debate has
ensued about whether testing positively for BRCA1, a genetic marker that
when present increases a woman's risk of developing breast and ovarian cancer, ought to be grounds enough for a doctor to recommend preventative or
"risk-reducing" surgery on otherwise healthy bodies. Jolie's mother died of
cancer at only fifty-six years of age. Presumably, Jolie was well versed in statistical probabilities associated with the likelihood that she, too, would suffer
a similar fate. For many women in Jolie's predicament, personal experience
and statistical probabilities are the only evidences they have to go on. I invoke
the Angelina Jolie effect here not as an endorsement of her choice but to draw
readers' attention to the complexity of weighing evidence against perceptions
of risk when making medical decisions.

Regardless of how readers view Jolie's (no doubt privileged) choice to
undergo preventative surgeries, her assertion about how cancer evokes a
"deep sense of powerlessness" likely resonates among readers from every

socioeconomic status. The powerlessness caused by cancer is pervasive. Genetic biomarkers, statistical analyses of survival, and characterizations such as "best practice" or "standard of care" are used routinely in cancer care, but are, by and large, mysteries to those who are unfamiliar with such specialized practices and discourses. We can assume that, in conversations with her doctor, Jolie was provided with accurate and useful information about her diagnosis, prognosis, and options for treatment. *Bodies in Flux* augments and perhaps supplements such private, doctor-patient conversations and attends to the methodological materiality associated with doing evidence-based cancer care. Mindful of the millions of people who live in a persistent state of prognosis (Jain 2013), I highlight how, in evidence-based medicine, methods materialize matter in meaningful ways.

After nearly a decade of studying evidential construction in the biomedical backstage, I have identified four specific methods with which medical professionals attune to corporeal flux in cancer care: evidential visualization, assessment, synthesis, and computation. To illustrate, consider the backstage, material-discursive labor that had to take place prior to my uncle's official cancer diagnosis. First, his disease was *visualized*. To do this, doctors worked with a host of technologies to capture, quantify, and interpret my uncle's body data (e.g., tumor size and placement, additional health concerns, comorbidities). Second, medical professionals *assessed* these body data. They relied on statistical calculations of survival by comparing previous patients' experiences to my uncle's unique disease experiences. Third, doctors reasoned about possible prognoses and treatment options by invoking standardized guidelines—guidelines that were produced from *syntheses* of previous patients' body data. And to better understand the genetic complexities of life-threatening diseases like my uncle's, medical professionals perform *computational analyses* of similar patients' DNA. By the time any of these evidences are "accommodated" to patients and their care networks (Fahnestock 1986), details surrounding the material-discursive design work I just described are black-boxed (Latour 1987). For Latour, "black box" is a construct "used by cyberneticians whenever a piece of machinery or a set of commands is too complex" (2–3). Black boxes collapse complexity into mere input and output. Black boxes coalesce disorder into something that "resembles an organised whole.... When many elements are made to act as one, this is what I will now call a black box" (Latour 1987, 131). *Bodies in Flux* props open such cancer-care black boxes. It unearths scientific methods that are used to make evidence matter and mean in the biomedical backstage.

Over the last three decades, the phrase "evidence-based medicine" has become a discursive marker for rigor and reliability in biomedical practice. Specifically, evidence-based medicine is defined as "the conscientious, explicit, and judicious use of current best evidence to guide decisions about patient care" (Sackett et al. 1996, 71). Before the practice was referred to as evidence-based medicine, randomized and well-controlled clinical trials were called critical appraisals. When Gordon Guyatt made programmatic changes to McMaster University's medical school in the 1990s, he advocated for educational instruction and practices that placed proven evidence (as could be supported through critical appraisals) ahead of experts' authoritative experiences and opinions. Critical appraisals acted as guidebooks by granting practitioners a sense of randomized trials' methodological rigor. Guyatt's revisions meant that methodological rigor now trumped clinical expertise. Evidence-based medicine soon displaced expert-based medicine, and young physicians who embraced randomized controlled trials' methodological superiority and evidential authority soon found themselves empowered.[1]

While some regard evidence-based medicine as a recent phenomenon concomitant with so-called scientific progress, for reasons I will soon describe in greater detail, I argue that medical practice has always been evidence based. Evidence-based medicine is not just an insistence on using evidence to make decisions. Medical practitioners have for centuries used evidence to make decisions. Rather, implicit in the era of evidence-based medicine is an agreement among contemporary medical practitioners that *methods matter*. That is, evidential worthiness and weight in modern-day biomedical practice hinges on methodological transparency and quality.

To demonstrate that contemporary evidence-based medical decision making is just as complicated as it ever was, scholars from various disciplines have sought to account for the role of affect, logic, intuition, persuasion, and experiential knowledge in medical practice (see, e.g., Denney 1999; Derkatch 2008; Graham 2011; Grossman and Leach 2008; Lambert 2006; Little et al. 2002; Mykhalovskiy and Weir 2004). Some scholars (in particular, those who characterize their work as medical rhetoric) have conducted important research about how evidence and expertise are leveraged during decision making (e.g., Charon and Wyer 2008; Derkatch 2008; Graham and Herndl 2013; Hikins and Cherwitz 2011; Majdik and Keith 2011; Schryer et al. 2009). But what do we know about the rhetorical design of medical evidences, themselves? What are medical evidences' material-discursive lineages? Until now, methods by which evidence is visualized, assessed, synthesized, and computed *prior to* the deliberative decision-making moment have garnered little attention from medical rhetoricians and technical communicators. While scholars in medical rhetoric (myself included) have conscientiously pored over transcripts from impassioned doctor-patient interactions and pharmaceutical policy deliberations, we have remained largely unfamiliar with (if not ignorant of) the evincing methods with and on which those conversations and deliberations are predicated.

As we seek answers to questions about whose evidence counts and what counts as evidence, methods for making biomedical evidence meaningful invite if not require constant critical attention. Examining methods with which medical professionals design evidence draws attention to and demystifies but also makes strange modern medicine's prophetic practices. As objects of study, scientific methods for navigating medical uncertainty are complex processes of becoming (Bohm 1981). Human, nonhuman, and computational actors collaboratively design the evidence with which decisions are later made. Understanding how evidential materials do rhetorical work in the biomedical backstage—specifically, how visuals evince, and how evidences are then assessed, synthesized, and computed—makes for more informed and agential patients, technical communicators, and participants during individual and public policy decision making. I argue that the material-discursive labor required to elevate quotidian biological processes to evidential status is not merely epiphenomenal to acts of diagnosis, treatment, and prognosis.

So, how does backstage, invisible design work render the argumentative grounds on which a medical decision may be made? To answer this question, each chapter props open the following biomedical, backstage black boxes: pathologists' and radiologists' methods for imaging cancer; policy makers' statistical methods for assessing survival probabilities; oncologists' methods for synthesizing evidence so that cancer-screening protocols can be established; and direct-to-consumer genetic testing companies' computational methods for commoditizing health futures. Examinations of scientific methods for negotiating medical uncertainty build on what Latour (1987) calls contexts of discovery, or science in the making. In each case study, I explore how human, nonhuman, and computational collaborations shape evidences that inform medical decisions—decisions that help to allay the deep sense of powerlessness often bred by the threat of disease and diagnostic uncertainty. Understanding this labor is important if medical professionals truly value shared or patient-centered decision making (cf. Charles et al. 1997, 1999). And since multiple publics are increasingly incorporated into democratic decision making about medical and scientific policies, a rich understanding of how evidences are rhetorical constructions might help lessen the degree to which the specter of error-free, scientific objectivity presides over such deliberative events. Finally, disclosing the rhetorical underpinnings of how medical professionals create diagnostic and prognostic order from biomedical chaos might help to advance nuanced definitions for and practices of care (cf. Mol, Moser, and Pols 2010).

## EVIDENTIAL MATTERS BY WAY OF THE TUMOR BOARD

As readers are probably already well aware, cancer care requires collaboration across many fields of expertise. It is not uncommon for a patient to have anywhere from five to ten doctors attending to her case at one time. To improve continuity of care across specialties, medical professionals meet regularly in behind-the-scenes meetings called tumor board conferences. During tumor board conferences, cancer-care professionals from a range of expertise discuss and deliberate about the complexity and contingency of a mutual patient's case.[2] Cases brought to the attention of the tumor board are particularly difficult for one reason or another: Perhaps a patient has several comorbidities or lacks the support network needed for the aggressive treatment their diagnosis requires. Perhaps a patient has more than one cancer, and her oncologist may be unsure about which cancer to treat first or more forcefully. Perhaps the standard of care for a patient's cancer suggests one particular treatment route, but the oncologist has a hunch that a different route might be more effective in this unique case. Because of cancer-care complexities like these, medical professionals will request that their patient's case be brought to the attention of their colleagues at a tumor board meeting. My interest in backstage evidential production and each of this book's analytic foci emerged inductively from a case study of tumor board meetings.

Inspired by David Olson's (1996) *World on Paper* and Christina Haas's doctoral seminar on literacy studies, I began the tumor board project in 2005 with a small-scale investigation of what I thought would be the role of the patient's chart in tumor board meetings. I was surprised to learn that the patient's physical chart was nowhere to be found during the deliberations I observed.[3] What *were* present during tumor board deliberations, however, were a host of evidences that medical professionals visually, textually, orally, and statistically displayed, described, and debated about. In the absence of a patient chart, each tumor board deliberator enacted a kind of in vivo presence of one or another form of evidence (e.g., the pathologist represented cellular evidences present in the patient's case, while the oncologist represented more personal evidences to be considered in the patient's case, such as the patient's mobility or the reliability of the patient's support system).

During every meeting I observed, the boardroom's lights were dimmed at a certain time and all attention was paid to the pathologist who displayed purple- and brown-colored renderings of tumor cells on a screen in the front of the room. From these renderings and the radiologist's visual displays of body data vis-à-vis positron emission tomography (PET), magnetic resonance imaging (MRI), and computed tomography (CT), medical professionals would infer certain biological processes and the presence (or not) of cancer.[4] Later in every meeting I observed, the tumor board chairperson (as was his role) invoked the most recent standard of care for the cancer diagnosis about which participants deliberated. I soon learned that standards of care relied on results from previously conducted clinical trials—results that have been synthesized into one, final recommendation. After the standard of care had been articulated, tumor board participants then deliberated about survival rates and expectations regarding a patient's quality of life should she choose one therapeutic option over another. During tumor board meetings, professional practice, previous experience, and individual expertise frequently collided. Discussions were heated. It soon became clear that—even without the presence of the patient's medical chart—tumor board meetings were a rich and dynamic context for rhetoricians and technical communicators to study how cancer care is practiced and performed.

Given tumor board meetings' genred nature (see Teston 2009), I traced and analyzed each meeting's deliberative process and identified exactly when an uncertainty or unknown was verbalized, as well as any and all evidences medical professionals invoked to resolve that uncertainty.[5] In an effort to mitigate what I now understand to be a body's indeterminacy (Barad 2003), deliberators most frequently invoked pathological and radiological images, statistically calculated survival data, and standards of care. Note that I use "indeterminacy," and not "uncertainty," to describe tumor board conundrums. I do so because casting the complexity of cancer care as uncertainty implies that there is or could be certitude. As readers will come to see in forthcoming case studies, certainty in cancer care is a bit of a fable. Bodies are in perpetual flux. Knowledge is always contingent.

Based on my observations of more than thirty patient case presentations during tumor board meetings, I can assert that the biomedical backstage is where medical professionals negotiate many of cancer care's contingencies. The biomedical backstage is limited to insiders (Goffman 1959) who "coconstruct" medical discourse and decisions (Barton 2004, 71). Each of the following chapters' analyses, therefore, are grounded investigations of what Gieryn (1999) and Latour (1987) call "upstream" evidential processes, or processes that predicate possibilities for future action.[6]

Tumor board meetings are a relatively recent strategy for navigating medical uncertainty; but medical professionals at least as far back as Plato have tried to methodically manage bodies in flux. In what follows, I argue not only that medical practice has always been evidence based, but I also highlight how those methods have always hinged on extrahuman, material-discursive phenomena.

## Premodern Medical Evidences

To divine medical futures, Plato, Aristotle, Cicero, and other ancients collaborated with the natural world. Of these, "oracles, dreams, divination by beasts and birds, and seeking the dead are the most celebrated" (Cohen 1964, 162). Sacrificial bodies were some of the earliest ways cultures attempted to navigate the unknown. Hepatoscopy (or the inspection of the liver of a sacrificial animal), consumption of the entrails of prophetic birds, and necromancy were premodern medical practitioners' methods for managing corporeal futures. Roman poet Marcus Annaeus Lucanus (39–65 A.D.) describes necromantic procedures whereby the knower would open a vein or bone of a corpse to bare the ghosts of the dead—ghosts that would then reveal both forensic and prophetic unknowns.

In an 1830 report intended to persuade the Massachusetts House of Representativeness to legalize the study of anatomy, it is written that, "the study of divination by sacrifices necessarily led to the study of anatomy of Animals, for it consisted in making observations while killing and cutting up the victim. These observations were not confined to external appearances, but were extended to the entrails and internal organization, and as these were found healthy or diseased, whole or defective, so was an inference drawn and the prediction ventured, for good or ill" (Massachusetts and Davis 1831, 7).

Divinations based on autopsy-like procedures such as these were often paired with methods of astrological contemplation. Etymologically, "contemplation" (*con* + *templation*) is derived from the act of constructing a diagram of the sky. This diagram was called a templum by Etruscan augurs (Cohen 1964, 173).[7] *Templums* (a word from which we derive "temple") were used to interpret systematically "the portens observed by the skywatcher" (Cohen 1964, 173). Scholars in uncertainty have since cataloged a host of premodern medical divination methods, including everything from alectronmancy (divining by way of a clucking cock) and cleromancy (divining by way of casting lots) to tyromancy (divining by way of the coagulation of cheese). Both Greek and medieval medicine's four humors—black and yellow bile, phlegm, and blood—were associated with the four seasons and astrological signs. Matter, movement, and time, therefore, formed the argumentative grounds on which premodern medical practitioners made evidence-based predictions.

While readers may be unfamiliar with such premodern material methods for managing medical indeterminacy, the following anecdote (author unknown) may resonate:

2000 B.C.—Here, eat this root.

1000 A.D.—That root is heathen. Here, say this prayer.

1850 A.D.—That prayer is superstition. Here, drink this potion.

1920 A.D.—That potion is snake oil. Here, swallow this pill.

1945 A.D.—That pill is ineffective. Here, take this penicillin.

1955 A.D.—Oops ... bugs mutated. Here, take this tetracycline.

1960-1999—39 more "oops." Here, take this more powerful antibiotic.

2000 A.D.—The bugs have won! Here, eat this root.

It is tempting to eschew premodern methods for managing medical uncertainty as based on little more than superstition. In his study of medical cuneiform texts, specifically the Babylonian *Diagnostic Handbook*, Heeßel (2004) disavows such a characterization: "The attempt to distinguish between magic and science or empiricism is considered to be a dead problem" (98). Specifically, he argues, "'Magic' and 'rationality' are modern categories by which western scholarship often distinguishes scientific and non-scientific attitudes. Seeking rational and magical elements in Babylonian medicine imposes modern values on it, and blurs the view of the mechanisms inherent within the Babylonian medical system itself. Indeed, dividing human thought processes into opposing principles such as 'magical' vs. 'scientific,' 'rational' vs. 'irrational' or 'primitive' vs. 'developed' characterizes structuralist approaches, and has been rightly criticized by Jack Goody who shows that this, as he calls it, 'Grand Dichotomy' is basically a-historic and obscures real development and change" (98). Heeßel and other medical historians honor as more than mere superstition the myriad methods by which the marrow of medical uncertainty was once sliced, diced, and carved away at.

In addition to methodically assessing flesh, phlegm, and other humors, premodern medical practitioners had methods for capturing and counting such corporeal evidences. Consider, for example, the pulse. Not only did the pulse mean different things among premodern medical practitioners, but it was also captured and measured differently. Kuriyama (1999), a historian of medicine who conducted a rich, oft-cited comparative cultural study of the history of Greek and Chinese medical traditions, explains that Chinese medical practitioners interpreted the pulse as signifying chi, or energy, whereas the

Greeks saw the pulse as evidence for anatomical function and efficiency.[8] Chinese medical practitioners' perspectives on the pulse are ultimately responsible for the "essential outlines of classical acupuncture" (Kuriyama 1999, 12). For Kuriyama (1999), that which separates an understanding of bodies as either musclemen or chi beings is "perceptual as well as theoretical" (13). Here, Kuriyama makes the very important move of insisting that Greek and Chinese medical practitioners' differing conclusions are not merely (or only) determined by varying theoretical understandings of a body in the West and the East. Instead, how a specific tradition comes to understand a body is conditioned by that tradition's methods for sensing, seeing, and touching. What the pulse signifies for Greek versus Chinese medical practitioners is a matter of evidential method, therefore. As Kuriyama (1999) puts it, "Theoretical preconceptions at once shaped and were shaped by the contours of haptic sensation" (60). It is not merely that "they felt it differently because they knew it differently" (60). Rather, for premodern medical practitioners, there is an ontological and epistemological partnership between knowing and sensing, making and being. Such partnerships persist still today (see Fountain 2014).

## Contemporary Medical Evidences

The tools and technologies with which contemporary biomedical professionals visualize, assess, synthesize, and compute evidence are certainly more designed than divined. But while contemporary medical wisdom appears more sophisticated, rational, and empirical than premodern methods for evidential design, medical professionals, scientists, and patients continue to grapple with the dubious nature of bodies in flux. Allopathic medicine's operating rooms and doctors' offices are inundated with a vast array of opportunities to see, touch, feel, and perceive bodies. Technologies for evincing bodies hang from doctors' office walls and around medical professionals' necks—always ready to hand. Evincing tools and technologies at once shape and are shaped by our diagnostic and prognostic traditions. Kim TallBear, Sheila Jasanoff, Donna Haraway, and other feminist theorists refer to the mutually constitutive relationship between phenomena and ways of knowing as coproduction or coconstitution. If material methods for evincing bodies in flux formulate the very grounds on which care can be practiced, attention to how medical evidence is visualized, assessed, synthesized, and computed is imperative. The technologies with which today's medical professionals amplify prognostic perception are as black-boxed and mysterious as ever before. As Weiser (1991) puts it: "The most profound technologies are those that disappear. They weave themselves into the fabric of everyday life until they are indistinguishable from it" (94). Perhaps more than any other evidential tradition, randomized and well-controlled clinical trials have woven themselves seamlessly into the fabric of contemporary biomedical practice.

## Clinical Trials

Medical professionals who rely on randomized, controlled clinical trials (RCTs) to make evidence-based decisions privilege methodological transparency, randomization, and experimental controls (see Marks [2000] for a much more detailed account of the prehistory of evidence-based medicine and the double blind clinical trial). Trial-based medical practices existed long before what is now referred to as evidence-based medicine (e.g., James Lind's controlled trial in 1747 that proved citrus fruit cures scurvy). Derkatch (2008) notes that because they are blinded, randomized, and reliant on placebos as controls, RCTs are imbued "with an ethos of disinterestedness" (372). The emergence of evidence-based medicine in general and the RCT specifically "sought to establish a new kind of medical practice based on evidence not eminence" (Derkatch 2008, 372). Contemporary biomedicine's methodical, systematic assessments and syntheses of evidence were inspired in part by a worldwide pharmaceutical catastrophe that resulted in the 1962 drug amendments. Post-thalidomide public outcry made necessary new, worldwide regulations that ensured pharmaceuticals would not be distributed without well-documented measures for assessing safety and efficacy.

It isn't always easy to document interventions' safety and efficacy, however. In *Bounding Biomedicine*, Derkatch (2016) argues that biomedicine's reliance on the scientific method, discursive standardizations, and rigorous evidential assessments are intended not just to maintain the boundaries of the profession but also to discredit the reliability and rigor of alternative medical therapies—therapies whose effectiveness (for a host of reasons) cannot be accounted for via RCTs. Derkatch (2008) invokes Porter's (1996) notion of what she calls the cult of impersonality to describe (again, what she calls) the nearly sacred status of evidence-based medicine's RCT. Yet, even as RCTs attempt to isolate the clinical effectiveness of a medical intervention from external actants that might influence results, there are always "social and cultural forces shaping research activities, the selection of evidences, and the resulting decisions and policies" (Lambert 2006, 2643). Indeed, we can never wholly shed human and nonhuman suasive actors from even the most well-designed and -executed RCTs.

## Algorithmic Protocols

One hallmark of contemporary biomedicine is the algorithmic protocol. The predictive power of algorithmic protocols lies in the assumption that body

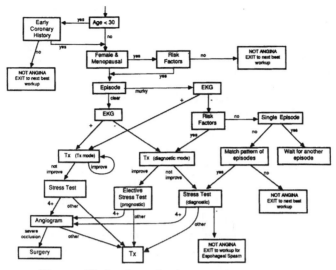

Figure 1.1 Workup for angina (source: Cohen et al. 1987)

data can be isolated from their environment. Algorithmic protocols such as standards of care, for example, are characterized as "a set of instructions" that "inform[s] the user what to do in a specified situation" (Berg 1998, 227). Based on the assumption that algorithmic protocols do more to silence noise than coconstruct an evidential signal, in the 1980s, the National Science Foundation (NSF) funded the development of a computer program called MUM (Management of Uncertainty in Medicine). This computer program enabled the NSF to use "control knowledge" when reasoning algorithmically about evidences' argumentative heft. As a result, medical professionals could use MUM to hypothesize about diagnoses. In the case of coronary artery disease, for example, MUM used the flowchart depicted in figure 1.1 to assess evidence in a way that maximized diagnostic accuracy at low cost.

Using hierarchical organization, assessment, and synthesis of the patient's age, medical history, sex, risk factors, and test results, MUM renders arguments presented linearly about diagnoses and treatment options for coronary artery disease. The development of this program exemplifies the rise of human and computational partnerships in evidence-based, biomedical practice. The "if this, then that" algorithmic aptitude of computational evidences like MUM stresses how visualization, assessment, synthesis, and computation are not just meticulous and methodical but also enthymematic.

Enthymematic approaches for harnessing and operationalizing evidence toward some final, care-giving end are perhaps best illustrated by standard of care documents. For every known cancer there is a standard for care. The

National Cancer Center Network engages in a series of ongoing evidential vetting practices, including collating current evidence, composing guidelines, deliberating about what new evidences need to be considered, revising said guidelines, and so on. Members of the network perform evidential vetting practices at least twice, but sometimes as many as four times, a year. Within each resultant standard of care document is an algorithmic protocol that quantifies network members' consensus about a particular protocol. Notably, standard of care documents are more akin to flowcharts than discursive reports of evidence-based recommendations (see Teston 2009, figs. 3 and 4). Berg (1998), citing Feinstein (1973), makes the case that because of the flowchart-like, branching structure of algorithmic protocols, "a clinician can now, at long last, specify the flow of logic in his reasoning, [so that he] can begin to achieve the reproducibility and standardization required for science" (227). Berg's analysis of how algorithmic protocols can shift patients' eligibility for treatment leads him to conclude that "the introduction of a protocol generates a propensity to refocus medical criteria on those elements which behave in predictable and easily traceable ways. The tool contains a predisposition to build *simple, robust worlds*, without too many interdependencies or weak spots where contingencies can leak back in" (243; italics in the original). Flowcharts help manage bodies in flux. But while algorithmic protocols may harness indeterminacy into manageable bits and bytes, they simultaneously flatten and sterilize the complexity of disease, the human body, and its "material effects and processes" (Edbauer 2005, 23). Simple, robust worlds are built with the assumption that certitude is possible. They're built assuming contingencies can be controlled. They're built with the hope that medicine can be managed. Yet, all is flux.

### METHODS AS EVIDENTIAL ATTUNEMENT

Biomedical evidences do rhetorical work. Long before biomedical evidences can be invoked as grounds for or against a particular way forward, however, backstage biomedical methods materialize some possibilities and not others. A particular method used to materialize a body in flux does not "simply transport the 'profound clinical experience and thought' of X; it *transforms* it" (Berg 1998, 244; italics in the original). More than tools, translation, or transport of a priori realities, medical evidences are performances enacted through or enlivened by backstage biomedical methods.

Ultimately, I argue that evidential methods in the biomedical backstage are ways of being attuned to (and with) indeterminacy. That is, evidential methods attune medical professionals to both a body in flux and the materiality of disease. Rickert (2013) defines attunement as that which "indicates one's disposition in the world, how one finds oneself embedded in a situation. This point needs emphasis: being so entangled, so caught up in the richness of the situation, an attunement is nothing subjective. It is neither inside nor outside, as Heidegger says, but 'the way of our being there with one another.' ... It results from the co-responsive and inclusive interaction that brings out both immersion (being with) and specificity (the way of our being there)" (9). Evidential potentialities—or the material manifestations of bodies in flux and disease—always already exist. Methods discipline matter in a way that makes evidential potentialities meaningful.

Methods matter in that they materialize and make evidence meaningful. Methods for evincing a body contribute to contexts of medical decision making in important ways. Extending Edbauer's, Phelps's, and Syverson's (1999) rich understanding of the role of context, Rickert (2013) argues that "the local environment is not just a passive stage for human activity but an integral, active element in its own right" (10). He invokes the Greek word *periechon*, meaning atmosphere, ambiance, or surroundings, to describe environments as "more than a neutral, objective stage on which human drama and activity play out" (9). More than a decade before Rickert (2013) illustrated ambient environments' agencies by describing the relationship between vineyards' soil type and the growth of grapes for wine (ix–x), McWhorter (1999) described the agency of dirt: all living things come "from the activity of that undifferentiated, much maligned stuff we call dirt" (167). Alaimo (2008) puts it this way: "Word, flesh, and dirt are no longer discrete" (256). Building from Rickert (2013), McWhorter (1999), and Alaimo (2008), I argue that backstage methods in which biomedical professionals engage in the quotidian work of coproducing evidential order from biological chaos are a kind of ontological soil for future action.

Backstage methods for visualizing, assessing, synthesizing, and computing evidence are ways of being with corporeal indeterminacy and attuning to bodies in flux. How pathologists, for example, dwell amid (and despite) the indeterminacy presented by biological processes invisible to the naked eye is a matter of attunement. Key to this argument is that attunement necessitates entanglements between human, nonhuman, and computational actors. Such entanglements or intra-actions (Barad 2003, 2007) create possibilities for sense making amid what appears to be little more than nonsense. Detecting cancer, seeing pre- and postoperative differences, and determining a pharmacological intervention's effectiveness are all a matter of evidential attunement.

Even while endorsing the work of other scholars in the field who emphasize that medical practice depends on rhetorical decision making by human actors, I add a new dimension to such analyses: the suasive potential of material things—ontological soil—that have either been overlooked or regarded only as epiphenomenal to acts of diagnosis, treatment, and prognosis. Indeed, the scientist makes meaningful the move from matter to evidence. But matter turned evidence is not mere material marionette enlivened by human manipulators' scientific strings.

Recall that the human pulse did something for Chinese medical practitioners that it did not do for Greek practitioners. As Kuriyama (1999) explains,

> What do we feel when we place our fingers on the wrist, and palpate the movements there? We say: the pulsing artery. What else could there be? Chinese doctors performing the same gesture, however, grasped a more complex reality. The finger placed lightly on the right wrist at the *cun* position, diagnosed the large intestines, while the finger next to it discerned the state of the stomach. Pressing harder these two fingers probed, respectively, the flourishing or decline of the lungs and spleen. Under each finger, then, doctors separated a superficial (*Fu*) site, felt near the body surface, from a sunken (*chen*) site deeper down. There were thus six pulses under the index, middle, and ring fingers, and twelve pulses on the two wrists combined. (25)

The coexistence of contemporary biomedicine's singular pulse with Chinese medicine's twelve is best understood in terms of what Mol (2002) calls multiple ontologies. Mol's notion of multiple ontologies requires that we shed perspectivalism and embrace the possibility that multiple performances of the same phenomenon coexist in meaningful ways. For Mol, realities are multiple in practice. In multiple ontological spaces, possibilities for negotiating contingencies and understanding bodies in flux are manifold. Indeed, "different conceptual schemes are going to produce very different versions of the world," but such conceptual schemes "do not *constitute* the world; they depict it. This difference is very significant" (Hekman 2008, 110). Matter persists at mattering. What we need, therefore, is "a way to talk about the materiality of the body as itself an active, sometimes recalcitrant, force" (Alaimo and Hekman 2008, 4). Different social and material contexts "allow different bodies to be called forth ... ontologies are always bound up and inseparable from the material world, not determined by it but not independent, either" (Harris and Robb 2012, 676). More specifically, "ontologies are materially constituted and materials are negotiated ontologically. There is never a clear gap between a material thing and a person's ontological engagement with it. ... To understand how the material and the ontological come into being, we must give space both to the physical qualities of the world and to the manner in which the world's agencies are transformed through its engagement with people" (Harris and Robb 2012, 677). The space that Harris and Robb reference here—a space where the world's agencies are transformed through its associations and engagements with humans—can be located in biomedical methods for evincing bodies in flux. Such methodological spaces can then be studied by observing how medical professionals attune evidentially.

In medical practice, methods for evidential attunement enact prognostic possibilities. Laboratories and other predeliberative spaces where biomedical matter is materialized are fertile sites for observing and studying assemblages of people, bodies, practices, and objects involved in cocreating (or maintaining) a sense of order from biological chaos. Latour and Woolgar (1986) argue that the very process of constructing scientific facts *"involves the use of certain devices whereby all traces of production are made extremely difficult to detect"* (176; italics in the original). Illich (1981) and, later, Lampland and Star (2009) might characterize such mostly invisible, ambient labor as shadow work. My aim is to make more apparent the shadow work that makes matter mean. Along the way, I am mindful of Alaimo and Hekman's (2008) observation that it is "nearly impossible" for "feminism to engage with medicine or science in innovative, productive, or affirmative ways" because "the only path available is the well-worn path of critique" (4). My hope is that the following investigations of shadow work forge a new path—one that renders a rich understanding of the human, nonhuman, and computational entanglements that enable evidential attunement and, subsequently, deliberative decision making.

Although technical communicators and rhetoricians are quite adept at understanding the role of the human in medical practice, we do not yet know how to account for the role of nonhuman agents, or things. Some readers may even find troubling the very notion of a nonhuman agent. After all, how could a nonhuman, or a thing, have agency? The answer to that question requires a book-length project of its own, and many scholars, some of whom characterize themselves as new materialists, have accomplished just that. (For a rhetorical perspective, see Barnett and Boyle's [2016] collection: *Rhetoric, Through Everyday Things*). Alaimo and Hekman (2008) argue that "nature is agentic—it acts, and those actions have consequences for both the human and nonhuman world" (5). Moreover, "we need ways of understanding the agency, significance, and ongoing transformative power of the world—ways that account for myriad 'intra-actions' (in Karen Barad's terms) between phenomena that are material, discursive, human, more-than-human, corporeal, and technological" (5). Barnett and Boyle (2016) similarly remind readers that much of new materialist and object-oriented scholarship is born of Heidegger's essay, "The Thing." Said simply: Things connect. Things *do*.

The so-called new materialist and nonhuman turn does not necessarily "deny individual agency or cognition" to humans; rather, it deemphasizes the role of "individual human beings to avoid overdetermining human agency and underdetermining roles played by other parts of the system" (McNely, Spinuzzi, and Teston 2015, 4). The methodological move to consider ontological whole or oneness (Bennett 2010) within which evidential labor is accomplished requires attention to shadow work—the very kind of backstage, scientific methods for navigating medical indeterminacy I examine in forthcoming chapters. Previously, shadow work may have been thought of only as epiphenomenal to broader activities of which they are a part. Extending Latour's constructs, "actant" and "network effect," Bennett (2010) draws our attention to material agencies, or "effectivity of nonhuman or not-quite-human things" (ix). Contrary to seeing technologies and other nonhumans as mediational in a Vygotskian sense, new materialists argue that matter (including space, time, and space-time) matters well enough on its own, mediation notwithstanding. Similarly, Callon, Lascoumes, and Barthe (2009) argue that obscure work, instruments, and disciplined bodies participate in networked activities "*in their own right*" (57; italics in the original). Although some have called this brand of materialism new, others (i.e., those who align themselves with material feminists) would suggest there is nothing *new* at all about this materialism.[9]

Indeed, prior to the new materialist turn, many Indigenous scholars argued for increased attention or at least a greater understanding of associations between human and nonhuman agents. Hekman (2008) notes that "one of the most radical elements of Latour's theory is his assertion that nonhuman entities *act*" (93; italics in the original). Humans and nonhumans make up a "collective that involves the exchange of human and nonhuman properties inside a corporate body" (Hekman 2008, 93). Latour's collective is quite akin to Pickering's (1995) mangle: "The world makes us in the same process by which we make the world" (Pickering, quoted in Hekman 2008, 94). Some readers might be more familiar with how Deleuze and Guattari (1987) theorize human-nonhuman associations. Their construct for such associations is assemblage: "An assemblage, in its multiplicity necessarily acts on semiotic flows, material flows, and social flows simultaneously" (quoted in Hekman 2008, 100). For Deleuze and Guattari (1987), observable results from assemblages' multiplicities reside at the seat of "practice." In this book, I locate material-discursive intra-actions between humans and nonhumans at the seat of method.

Understanding associations between human and nonhuman agents invites us to recognize that *things* in medical practice *do work*, and medical professionals do work with them. Braidotti (2013) describes this as "co-presence," or "the simultaneity of being in the world together"—an assertion that has "important implications for the production of scientific knowledge" (169). Posthumanist scholars argue that, in fact, we have never truly been fully or independently human. That is, "the human has always coevolved, coexisted, or collaborated with the nonhuman" (Grusin 2015, x). Humans have always done work with "the generative force of a generative universe," or what Braidotti (2013), citing Guattari (1995), refers to as "'chaosmosis,' which is nonhuman and in constant flux" (170). It follows, then, that bodies are neither "pure culture" nor "pure biology" (Grosz 1994, 191). Evidential attunement in biomedical practice is not an exclusively human enterprise; it results from a series of methodical performances that emerge from human and nonhuman partnerships.[10]

### KEY ANALYTIC CONCEPTS

Several analytic constructs guide how I understand evidential attunement in the biomedical backstage. First, in addition to Illich's (1981) shadow work and Rickert's (2013) ambient attunement, forthcoming chapters also rely on Barad's (2007) understanding of how matter and meaning are entangled. Her construct, intra-action—which she describes as "a profound conceptual shift in our understanding of causality" (333)—helps shed light on the biomedical and corporeal consequences of human-nonhuman partnerships in medical practice (cf. Gries's [2015] notion of "distributed causality"). Barad argues, "It is through specific agential intra-actions that the boundaries and properties of the 'components' of phenomena become determinate and that particular material articulations of the world become meaningful" (333). My use of "material-discursive" as a descriptor for the kind of labor or rhetorical design work that co-occurs in the biomedical backstage has its roots in Barad's (2003) notion of agential realism. That is, when I use "material-discursive," I am highlighting how "apparatuses are specific material practices through which local semantic and ontological determinacy are intra-actively enacted" (Barad 2003, 820). Said another way: things and the words used to describe them are mutually constitutive. In fact, Barad (2003) posits that "outside of particular agential intra-actions, 'words' and 'things' are indeterminate," and "both materiality and discursive practices are rethought in terms of intra-activity" (820). When I mobilize "material-discursive" I affirm Hekman's (2008) argument that "what we need now is not a theory that ignores language as modernism did, but rather a more complex theory that incorporates language, materiality, and technology into the question" (92). Material-discursive methods for evidencing disease mark the space where meaningful and consequential intra-actions occur. Evidential methods provide a set of observable practices that rhetoricians can explore to learn about how medical professionals attune to bodies in constant flux.

Second, theories about the suasive potential of things in the biomedical backstage—for example, stains, slides, and scopes in the next chapter—are motivated by Bennett's (2010) radical suggestion that we should acknowledge the agency or vitality of nonhuman or not-quite-human things. Bennett makes the case that rejecting anthropomorphism "is bound up with a hubristic demand that only humans and God can bear any traces of creative agency" (120). For Bennett, understanding nonhuman actants' agency is inherently political. That is, how we view events of social consequence might actually change "if we gave the force of things more due" (Bennett 2010, viii). Alaimo and Hekman (2008) make a similar case: "Political decisions are scripted onto material bodies; these scripts have consequences that demand a political response on the part of those whose bodies are scripted" (8). In *Bodies in Flux*, therefore, Bennett's (2010) notion of vibrant matter informs how I understand the political and ethical implications of working alongside extra-human agential forces when making claims about bodily being.

Third, concomitant with forthcoming chapters' reconsideration of who and what has agency in the biomedical backstage is a deliberate effort to shed reductive theories about what, exactly, rhetoric is and does. Specifically, I take to be true Rickert's (2013) assertion that "rhetoric cannot be reduced to the intent—deliberate or posited—to persuade" (160). Echoing Edbauer's (2005) ecological view of rhetoric, Rickert (2013) makes the case that studying and doing rhetoric requires attention to "the larger background, including our activity against which the particular assemblage of elements comes to be seen as suasive" (160). Evidential assemblages and enmeshments, therefore, shed light on what (it) *is*. As Rickert (2013) argues, "Language, person, and environment, then, are perhaps not so much *linked*, and from such a linkage established as coadaptive, as they are enmeshed and enfolded, making them mutually conditioning entities that have already emerged from a larger, worldly whole. From this ambient perspective, the privilege that we typically accord human agency in the world is dimmed so that we see anew what human-centered thought too often places in shadow" (106). The following chapters invite readers to dim "the privilege that we typically accord human agency" (Rickert 2013, 106) and to account for shadow work, or behind-the-scenes, rhetorical labor—labor that Rickert (2013) might call "a stitchwork of material, practical, and discursive relations by which any work at all can be conducted" (93). Along the way, I mobilize biomedicine's evidential assemblages and animate anew key concepts in rhetorical theory, including *kairos*; enthymeme; stases; Toulminian grounds, warrants, and backing; boundary objects and infrastructures; and *phronesis*. In so doing, I hope to demonstrate for readers the explanatory power of both classical and contemporary rhetorical theory in technical, scientific, and medical contexts.

## OBJECTS OF ANALYSES

The investigative sites (e.g., pathology laboratories and Food and Drug Administration pharmaceutical hearings) and methodological practices (e.g., statistical analyses and genetic sequencing) that I examine in *Bodies in Flux* point to places where key stakeholders wade collaboratively through a morass of medical indeterminacy and eventually arrive at cancer diagnoses, public policy decisions, treatment options, and quantifications of risk. These are sites and practices in which, while constructing possibilities for future action, matter and bodies "have a peculiar and distinctive kind of agency" (Frost 2011, 70). Because attempts at managing medical uncertainty in biomedical contexts take place between both human actors (e.g., doctors and their patients) and human and nonhuman actors (e.g., pathologists and microscopes), I posit theories about how evidential technologies such as hematoxylin and eosin stains, inferential statistics, and clinically meaningful endpoints are more than mere tools used by humans to find answers; evidential technologies such as these exert suasive force when possibilities for cancer care are made to matter. Each chapter's case study takes to be true Barad's (2007) notion of matter as an "active participant in the world's becoming" (803) and, as such, asks readers to be attentive to more than medicine's textual or linguistic representations. Analytic attention is on the messy, collaborative, and yet methodical practice of evidential visualization, assessment, synthesis, and computation.

I have chosen evidential visualization, assessment, synthesis, and computation not to elide other important practices involved in making medical decisions but to capture the complexity of medical decision making's pre-deliberative, backstage labor. Ultimately, methods for evidential design, such as medical imaging, inferential statistical analyses, meta-analyses of hundreds of published and unpublished clinical trial results, and using algorithms to pattern match genetic data, are argumentative grounds on which claims about cancer care are made. Understanding how medical professionals attune evidentially to bodies in flux sheds light not just on how to do rhetoric and how rhetoric does the world. Understanding how medical professionals attune evidentially to bodies in flux also forces us to consider the ethics of dwelling with disease, since as Audre Lorde (1980) wrote: "There must be some way to integrate death into living, neither ignoring it nor giving in to it" (13).

Furthermore, the patient-centered care that medical institutions like the Mayo Clinic espouse is founded on the assumption that doctors and patients engage in shared decision making. The Institute of Medicine defines patient-centered care as: "Providing care that is respectful of and responsive to individual patient preferences, needs, and values, and ensuring that patient values guide all decision-making" (Institute of Medicine 2001, 3). Patient-centered care assumes the patient is necessarily informed. However, what could be more black-boxed than the $p$ values that cancer researchers use to determine a treatment's efficacy? And the distinction between discipline-specific language like "progression-free survival" and "overall survival" (measures by which medical professionals assess medical interventions) is also a mystery to most. Cochrane systematic reviews (reports that are akin to meta-analyses of all previously published scientific findings) are rarely recognized as resources for patients who, for example, might be curious about the efficacy of cannabinoids for controlling chemotherapy-induced nausea and vomiting. And geneticists themselves now freely confess that they have more computed genetic data than they know how to use or what to do with. If there is any hope of abandoning a care model that conceals more than it reveals (either inadvertently or purposefully), discipline-specific evidential visualizations, assessments, syntheses, and computations deserve explication.

To clarify, I am not suggesting that patients and their care networks must, amid all else, become experts in biomedical evidences. Rather, I hope this book helps to unearth reasons for how and why it is that cancer care is not and could never be an objective science. Nor am I suggesting that there is something inherently deceptive about biomedical black boxes. Black boxes are essential to cancer care. Black boxes do the hard work of stabilizing, qualifying, and mobilizing "future use of ideas and facts" while aggregating and materializing alliances (Danius 2002, 41–42). Rhetorical analyses of the biomedical backstage's black boxes help map the sociotechnical alliances that greatly if not gravely affect the lives of patients, policy makers, and care workers themselves.[11] If nothing else, I hope to demonstrate rhetorical theory's explanatory power inasmuch as it helps bore a hole in medical practice's technological and scientific complexity.

In an age when many (but certainly not all) citizens are armed with an abundance of health information in online and other quotidian spaces, I make a case for medical practice and cancer care as a matter of evidential attunement. Access to symptom checkers, medical records, and online, algorithmic diagnostic tools does only so much in the way of democratizing medical data, managing medical uncertainty, and sharing decision making. After providing scholars, scientists, and everyday citizens an opportunity to peer into cancer care's biomedical backstage, I ultimately claim that medical practice is more than art or science. Medical practice involves a series of rhetorical negotiations that require *phronesis*, or practical wisdom.

### CASE STUDIES

Although others have attended to how medical or scientific images are rhetorical (e.g., Buehl 2016; Cartright 1995; Dumit 2004; van Dijck 2005), few have explicated the material-discursive and human/nonhuman methods for rendering medical images as evidence in the first place. Chapter 2, therefore, details how a body is evidenced through a series of visualization techniques. I ask: How do pathologists, pictures, stains, and scopes work together to evince whether (and if so, to what degree) cancer has become a part of a patient's body? Chapter 2 describes the obscure work, instruments, and disciplined bodies (Callon, Lascoumes, and Barthe 2009, 57) that materially evidence the corporeality of a person with cancer. Drawing on data from a previous study of medical professionals' visualization techniques and technologies (Teston 2012b), I animate anew the rhetorical construct, *kairos*, as a skill necessary for attuning to molecular and cellular phenomena, or that which is in a constant state of flux.

The probability of survival for a person newly diagnosed with cancer is contingent on their options for and decision about treatment. But how are those options rendered possible in the first place? What kind of material-discursive labor warrants an oncologist's treatment recommendation? I explore these questions in chapter 3 and report results from a study of how medical statisticians, pharmaceutical companies, policy makers, and cancer researchers use inferential statistics to assess survival data. Statistical assessments act as argumentative warrants for patients' treatment options. This method for evidential assessment, therefore, lays the groundwork for predictions about a patient's survival probability. In addition to accommodating discipline-specific details of survival analysis and inferential statistics for readers without expertise in either area, I highlight, in chapter 3, how disease experiences that could very well affect a patient's treatment options are sometimes silenced by current methods for evidential assessment. To do this, I report on analyses of how one large, regulatory network—the Food and Drug Administration—uses Kaplan-Meier survival curves, hazard rates, confidence intervals, effect size, and $p$ values to assess evidence. Using rhetorical theory as an analytic lens helps to unpack the suasive properties of inferential statistics. I theorize probabilistic reasoning in general as *poesis* and inferential statistics in particular as enthymematic and argue that suasive properties of inferential statistics, such as hazard rates, confidence intervals, effect size, and $p$ values, formulate a chain of premises that permit probabilistic arguments. Furthermore, I describe how each enthymematic premise attunes deliberators to data in such a way that some forms of evidence are deemed more (or less) meaningful than others. Chapter 3 concludes by imagining how biomedical practitioners might power assessment methods in ways that are more capable of valuing evidences that resist quantification.

Since results from clinical trials are grounds on which medical professionals make recommendations for cancer care, chapter 4 explores how medical professionals synthesize clinical trial evidences toward some final argument or clinical recommendation. The specific variety of evidential synthesis I analyze—the Cochrane Systematic Review (CSR)—makes some data about cancer care more authoritative than others. The CSR not only functions as a stabilized-for-now (Schryer 1993; Spinuzzi 2003; Teston 2009) set of guidelines that grant expert medical ethos to researchers and clinicians who follow the CSR's recommendations, but they also act as decision-making heuristics on a more local level. That is, CSRs can inform how decision aids are developed and designed for real-time clinical encounters between a doctor and her patient. Cochrane Systematic Reviews provide comprehensive commentary about the current state of knowledge while promoting probabilistic possibilities. To better understand Cochrane reviewers' reasoning when synthesizing evidence into a final argument, I report on results of a modified Toulminian analysis of a representative sample of CSRs. Noting that Cochrane reviewers exclude more data than they include in their CSRs (a rhetorical practice I refer to as evidential cutting), I pair Toulmin's model for argumentation with stasis theory to perform an innovative analysis of how CSR authors make decisions about evidential cuts. Chapter 4 concludes with a call to action: I argue for increased collaboration between technical communicators, rhetoricians, and medical scientists when designing clinical trials so that qualitative evidences might be better integrated into evidential syntheses.

Inspired by the Obama administration's promise of precision medicine and the recent proliferation of genetic testing as an attempt to manage biomedical flux, in chapter 5 I argue for constant critical attention to emerging methods for evidential attunement. One emergent method for attuning evidentially is direct-to-consumer genetic testing. Methods for direct-to-consumer genetic sequencing black-box medical data in precarious ways (see Teston [2016] for more on precarity in medical practice). I explore two direct-to-consumer genetic testing companies' precarious practices by using

Clarke's (2005) situational mapping method and I reframe at-home genetic tests through the theoretical lenses of posthumanism, feminist technoscience, and Illichian shadow work. Chapter 5 offers a material-discursive critique of genetic sequencing's boundary work, or what I call (building off of chapter 4's findings) computational cut making. Under the rubric of boundary work, genetic mutation is a malleable discursive phenomenon—*not* a stable and secure material fact. The chapter concludes with a critique of precision medicine's individualistic narratives of biomedical choice, autonomy, and empowerment. Chapter 6, the concluding chapter of *Bodies in Flux*, makes a case for medical practice as *phronesis* and invites readers to consider what it might look like to dwell with rather than attempt to fight against cancer.

I take seriously Mol, Moser, and Pols's (2010) assertion that "good care" in medicine is "persistent tinkering in a world full of complex ambivalence and shifting tensions" (14). Entrée into backstage biomedical tinkering practices prepares readers for the inevitability of tough decisions no doubt to come. I hope that providing details about how, exactly, cancer care is an act of rhetorical negotiation helps lessen the weight of medical decision making's argumentative armor. Certainty is simply not possible. Rather than a book of prescriptions for improving health care based on ex cathedra rhetorical scrutiny, *Bodies in Flux*'s fine-grained analyses contribute to ongoing conversations about how humans and nonhumans coconstruct and compute a sense of certainty when it is most elusive.

# 2. EVIDENCING VISUALS

*This study does not try to chase away*
*doubt but seeks instead to raise it.*
Annemarie Mol, *The Body Multiple*

KALEIDOSCOPE
*In small lights*
*darting off a prism*
*or a glass*
*of low proportions*
*the world comes back to me.*
*Its yellow far from red*
*and green from blue.*
*Shining only when*
*in shards*
*it gives a partial view.*

Sylvia Scribner, from
*Mind and Social Practice*

Bodies are in perpetual flux—especially at the cellular level. Scientists estimate that a single human body contains 37.2 trillion cells (Bianconi et al. 2013), and of these trillions of cells approximately 300 million of them die every single minute.[1] In rapid fashion, as some cells die, others replicate. When we consider such numbers within the context of a cancer diagnosis, the significance of cellular flux is even more startling. One researcher estimates that a one-centimeter breast cancer tumor sheds, on average, three million cells per day (Lee et al. 2013, 196). The rapid rate at which cancerous cells are shed into the bloodstream "provides a lot of opportunities for spreading into other organs" (Lee et al. 2013, 196). Here we see how important it is to understand biological bodies as agential. That is, "biological entities" are "complex and ever-transforming" and "are neither passive nor mechanistically determined" (Alaimo 2008, 245). Rather, biological entities or cellular phenomena "exhibit '*active* response to change and contingency'" (Birke, quoted in Alaimo 2008, 245).

The type of brain cancer that took the life of Stephen P. Witte—the man who founded the doctoral program from which I graduated and whose work is formative to the thinking of many in my field—is said to grow so quickly that many die within one year, and 90 percent of patients die after three years. When it comes to cancer care, matter, movement, and time intra-act in awful and precarious ways. This chapter sets the stage for investigations of how we attune rhetorically (Rickert 2013) to matter, movement, and time in cancer care. Specifically, I focus on scientific methods for attuning visually, and ask: Through what backstage biomedical methods do cancer-care professionals negotiate constant cellular and molecular change?

Sight is and always has been central to evidence-based medical practice. In premodern medicine, Chinese medical practitioners had "faith in visual knowledge" (Kuriyama 1999, 153) for the ways variations in color could evince the waxing and waning of an illness: "Wang er zhi zhi—to gaze and know things, the pinnacle of medical acumen—was thus to know things before they had taken form, to grasp 'what is there and yet not there.' As an illness becomes more serious, its corresponding color intensifies. If the color fades 'like clouds completely dispersing (yun chesan),' the illness will soon pass. One observes whether the color is superficial or sunken to know the depth of the illness, whether the color is dispersed or concentrated to know the proximity of crises" (179). Over time and in collaboration with a host of nonhuman and not-quite-human objects contemporary biomedical practitioners attune themselves to biological or molecular phenomena and, based on those attunements, medical professionals make inferences about evidences' meaning within the context of a particular patient's unique cancer-care scenario.[2]

Herein lies the rub, however: in the time it takes to visually evince disease, the evidential artifact itself becomes a kind of relic. Biomedical practitioners have no choice in the matter. They are forced to give objects their due (Marback 2008). The laboratory's time collides precariously with cancer's time. Evidential visualizations make it possible to see the spread of disease, but medical images can only account for that which has already happened. It seems as though we may never be able to keep up with a body in flux. Left in the wake of cellular replication, shedding, and death, however, are a series of meaningful intra-actional traces that mark what was at one time and place.

This chapter is motivated, therefore, by the following questions: What is the role of matter, movement, and time in evidencing a body visually? And how do time and cellular change affect what medical professionals can know about cancer diagnoses and prognoses? To explore these questions, I rely on the real-time, decision-making complexity associated with three patients' cancer-care presentations—those of Clarice, Sadie, and Monika. Alongside interviews with a pathologist and an oncologist, analyses of how tumor board deliberators grapple with the complexity of caring for these three women afford insights into how we might mobilize *kairos* as a rhetorical skill necessary for negotiating medical uncertainty. But first, to provide readers with a sense of the biomedical backstage from which forthcoming analyses of visuals-as-evidence derive, below is a snapshot of one tumor board meeting.

## The Tumor Board: A Snapshot

It is 11:54 A.M. on Wednesday; men and women in white coats gradually flood into the River East's Hospital Boardroom (this and all other names are pseudonyms to be in compliance with my institution's Human Subjects Research Institutional Review Board). Two older, retired oncological surgeons stand in front of a bowl of ice and stacks of soda speaking in Spanish to one another while the tumor board chairperson fills his plate with the pharmaceutical company–sponsored lunch. Radiologists, oncologists, pathologists, oncological nurses, medical students, and other medical professionals are seated at the table with their lunches while reviewing the tumor board participant packet cover sheet to find out which two cases will be presented. At 12:00 P.M., the tumor board chairperson, who is an oncologist, quickly reviews a series of standard, required disclaimers: "We are teleconferencing this afternoon with River West Hospital. Just a reminder that you must fill out the blue CME [continued medical education] form in order to get credit for being here—and please provide comments as you see fit so we can do things better in the future. Also, everything discussed or mentioned here today has been approved by the FDA. Oh and today's lunch is provided by Pfizer Corporation." The oncologist to his left nods, clears his throat, and begins to describe his patient's relevant background information. After this brief sixty-second introduction to the patient and her relevant medical background he ends with, "so she goes to see the surgeon, and prior to the biopsy the PET scan shows . . ." Almost on cue, an administrative assistant in the room gets up and dims the lights, and the radiologist who sits across the table from the oncologist displays a black-and-white image of a skeleton with a bright red hotspot in the center of its chest.

*

Tumor board debates are concerned primarily with how to treat patients now and moving forward (i.e., what to do tomorrow, next week, next month, and thereafter). But before deliberators move to discussion about future action, the meeting begins with an introduction to the patient through basic information and details about what has already occurred in the patient's care. During this time, deliberators wade for a while in concerns of a forensic nature, and sometimes seek answers to such questions as, for example: Why was the patient prescribed estrogen for bone loss? Why did the patient undergo a vaginal hysterectomy instead of an abdominal hysterectomy? Once tumor board participants deal with inquiries and challenges of a forensic nature, pathologists and radiologists display images that indicate a cancer's most recent material conditions. From this point forward, deliberators move into heated debates that are frequently fraught with differences in expertise, background experience, and medical knowledge.

Interviews with medical professionals who participated in the tumor board provide a better sense of medical images' suasive properties. Before I present interview data, below I describe the grounded theory methodological approach I used to capture and analyze such data.

## Grounded Theory Methods

A grounded theory approach to data collection and analysis guides the research reported both here and in a previous account of a portion of this project (Teston 2012b). Grounded theory evolved out of Glaser and Strauss's three-year qualitative study of hospitals in the San Francisco Bay area in California. Specifically, the authors developed an "integrated theory about awareness contexts as they pertain to dying in hospitals" (Glaser and Strauss 1965, 286). Glaser and Strauss's grounded theory approach asks field-workers to "plunge into social settings where the important events about which they will develop theory" are going on "naturally" (288). This study's systematic approach and resultant substantive theories are similarly developed from grounded analyses of real-time observations, interviews, and conversations.

What is unique about a grounded theory approach is that "there tends to be blurring and intertwining of coding, data collection, and data analysis, from the beginning of the investigation until near its end" (Glaser and Strauss 1965, 288). In other words, the collection, coding, and analysis of data happen iteratively, or co-occur. This approach ensures that any substantive theory built as a result of said investigations are inductively derived from and closely resemble actual real-time happenings. With a grounded theory approach, data are not retrofitted into a predetermined theory. Rather, theories are built from, rather than about, data (see Farkas and Haas 2012). To do this, I performed a constant comparison method in which the happenings I observed were iteratively coded, categorized, and compared over two phases of grounded research.

In both research phases—data collection phases one and two—I relied on a series of inductively derived observational heuristics with $x$ and $y$ axes that allowed me to document real-time happenings (see Teston [2012a] for additional details about these observational heuristics), including participants, evidential references, and the passage of time. During phase one, which consisted of fourteen tumor board visits, observational heuristics were constantly modified to more systematically collect data about who the participants were, what they talked about, how they talked about subjects, and so on. Phase one, therefore, was dedicated to open coding, or what Strauss (1987) calls the "unrestricted coding of the data" that yields concepts and dimensions that are "entirely provisional" (28).

During data collection phase two, which lasted six weeks, categories were developed and saturated enough that I could use a single, stable, final observational heuristic to systematically collect data. This phase was dedicated mostly to what Strauss (1987) and Glaser and Strauss ([1967] 2007) called "theoretical sampling," or "a means 'whereby the analyst decides on analytic grounds what data to collect next and where to find them'" (Strauss 38). Phase two yielded the emergence of four major categories (based on patterns noted in observational heuristics) that were then mapped on to one another and onto the passage of time in minutes and seconds. This kind of mapping technique yielded a temporal and contextual trace of how tumor board deliberations unfolded.

## Early Findings

One of this study's major categories or findings was a record of the four modes through which tumor board members deliberated. Codes within this category included text, talk, gesture, and images. Of those four codes, I determined via observational heuristics that one of the primary ways medical professionals collaborate about their patients' future care is by invoking on-screen projections of medical images. In all eleven patient case presentations during data collection phase two, radiological and pathological images were presented on-screen and referenced orally numerous times. I coded references to radiological or pathological images as either of the following: (1) an oral reference to pathological and/or radiological image or (2) the visual display of one pathology or radiology image (with an accompanying oral description). So, for instance, if a pathologist displayed and described a series of four images rendered as a result of a particular staining technique, they were counted as four pathological/radiological image references.

In table 2.1, I provide details about the length (in minutes and seconds) of each patient case presentation and the total number of radiological and pathological references made during each patient case presentation. For example, in patient case presentation one, the deliberation was twelve minutes, and during those twelve minutes I documented ten radiological and pathological references. In sum, in each of the eleven patient case presentations I

**Table 2.1 Radiological-Pathological References and Total Time**

| Patient Case Presentation | Length (min:sec) | Radiological-Pathological References (Visual and Oral) | Total Time of Radiological-Pathological Presentation (min:sec) |
|---|---|---|---|
| 1 | 12:00 | 10[a] | 5:50 |
| 2 | 21:21 | 9 | 1:25 |
| 3 | 17:56 | 16 | 9:43 |
| 4 | 12:00 | 9 | 3:19 |
| 5 | 24:29 | 9 | 4:48 |
| 6 | 12:05 | 10 | 3:53 |
| 7 | 14:13 | 14 | 5:19 |
| 8 | 29:00 | 14 | 9:33 |
| 9[b] | 18:09 | 4 | 3:00 |
| 10 | 15:33 | 10 | 7:06 |
| 11 | 14:59 | 9 | 5:02 |

[a] Not including the five repeat displays due to technical difficulty.

[b] Patient case presentation 9 is an anomaly not only for this set of eleven presentations, but also for the fourteen presentations I observed in data collection phase 1. It is an anomaly because, during this tumor board meeting, participants were debating about why a patient they mutually shared recently passed away during a visit to the emergency room. In this incident, the tumor board meeting was more forensic than deliberative.

analyzed, radiological and pathological references were made a minimum of four times and as many as fourteen times, and they accounted for anywhere from a minute and a half of the total deliberation to approximately ten minutes of the deliberation. The longest patient case presentation was approximately thirty minutes while the shortest was twelve minutes. It was clear that visualizations of evidence occupy a good deal of the tumor board's deliberation.

After radiologists or pathologists present their evidence, medical professionals continue to reference orally the visual information throughout their deliberations. Table 2.2 shows specific temporal data on the point during deliberations at which radiological and pathological references (visual and oral) were made. In all patient case presentations, visual evidences occupy the tumor board's deliberations at least once, but as many as four distinct periods. For example, in patient case presentation ten, deliberators referenced and discussed visuals as evidence at one minute, forty-five seconds into their

## Table 2.2 Temporal Data Regarding Periods of References to Visual Evidences

*Temporal Data Regarding*
*References to Visual Evidences*

| Patient Case Presentation | Time Span (min:sec) | Specific References |
|---|---|---|
| 1 | 2:30–4:30 | 4 radiological |
|  | 4:30–6:30 | 5 pathological |
|  | 10:30–11:20 | 5 pathological |
| 2 | 2:20–3:45 | 3 radiological, 4 pathological |
| 3 | 2:01–3:14 | 3 radiological |
|  | 3:45–5:33 | 4 pathological |
|  | 6:26–9:34 | 4 pathological |
|  | 10:00–13:10 | 2 radiological, 2 pathological |
| 4 | 2:35–4:10 | 2 radiological, and 4 pathological |
|  | 4:46–5:40 | 1 radiological |
| 5 | 1:12–6:00 | 1 radiological, 7 pathological |
| 6 | 2:27–5:10 | 6 pathological |
|  | 5:50–7:00 | 2 radiological |
| 7 | 3:15–5:31 | 4 radiological |
|  | 5:16–8:19 | 8 pathological |
| 8 | 1:25–3:15 | 2 radiological |
|  | 3:20–4:03 | 1 radiological |
|  | 4:20–7:40 | 3 radiological |
|  | 7:56–11:36 | 4 pathological |
| 9 | 2:30–5:30 | 3 pathological |
| 10 | 1:45–3:23 | 2 radiological |
|  | 3:23–6:20 | 3 pathological |
|  | 6:45–9:00 | 3 pathological |
|  | 9:32–9:48 | 1 radiological |
| 11 | 0:20–2:53 | 3 radiological |
|  | 3:55–6:24 | 4 pathological |

debate, again at three minutes, twenty-three seconds, again at six minutes, forty-five seconds, and finally at nine minutes, thirty-two seconds. I provide these data to demonstrate how visual evidences are weaved meaningfully into the tumor board's deliberations. Only in three patient case presentations (two, five, and nine) did visual evidences occupy just one, single deliberative period (one of which was an anomalous patient case presentation in which deliberators met to discuss the death of a patient in an emergency room visit).

On the whole, the study's temporal data demonstrate how important visual evidences are to tumor board deliberations. Documenting when and how frequently specific kinds of evidence are referenced doesn't tell us much about the backstage, material methods for rendering such evidences suasive in the first place, however. Interviews and in-depth explorations of three patient case presentations provide additional details about how visual evidence's material characteristics (rendered in the pathology lab's backstage) ultimately shape that which deliberators could debate about. Options for future action are born from backstage, biomedical methods for attuning to cancer's change over time.

### CANCER CARE'S SUASIVE IMAGES

In every patient case presentation I witnessed, medical images consistently marked the move out of forensic debate and into decision making about future action. In a previous report of these data (Teston 2012b), I sought to identify medical images' suasive properties in order to have a better sense of how deliberators transition out of forensic concerns and into possibilities for future action. What follows is a complementary analysis: how images' properties and the ways they are materialized backstage well prior to the deliberative moment have as much of an effect on deliberative decision making as do tumor board deliberators' argumentative moves themselves.

Visualization techniques, due in part to varying methods for seeing (albeit partially), attune biomedical practitioners to a body's most invisible elements and processes.[3] Two techniques for attuning visually to disease during tumor board deliberations are radiological imaging and pathological imaging. Data from imaging techniques are quantified and described in a report, and, in the case of a cancer diagnosis, from these data, oncologists and patients can then make decisions about possibilities for future action.

In what follows, I present results from my interviews with both a pathologist whom I call Dr. Marco and an oncologist whom I call Dr. Thomas. My discussions with Dr. Marco and Dr. Thomas should prepare readers for considering matter, movement, and time as contributors to bodies in perpetual flux. In particular, readers should note how imaging techniques assist medical professionals with mapping complex relationships between patients' bodies and the seemingly chaotic nature of cancer's matter, movement, and change over time.

## Radiological Images

According to both Dr. Marco and Dr. Thomas, radiological images make possible the anatomical detection or confirmation of a tumor. Radiological images evince a body in flux by providing information about the size and location of a tumor and where it has spread. Dr. Thomas notes that surgeons will frequently use radiological images of the patient's cancer as a guide when performing a biopsy. A biopsy involves the removal of a small tissue sample in or surrounding an area of the body that is cause for concern. In this instance, images act as corporeal maps for surgeons as they seek to gather navigational evidence without causing harm to surrounding tissue. Dr. Thomas also reports that he often orders X-rays, computed axial tomography (CT) scans, or magnetic imaging resonance (MRI) scans after a patient has undergone cancer treatment to determine if the cancer has responded to an oncological intervention. Through comparisons of postintervention scans with preintervention scans, medical images evince change over time.

Specifically, through intra-acting lenses and light, MRI scans create colorful contrasts and distinctions between otherwise indistinct corporeal conditions. These scans attune medical professionals to bodies in the following way:

> The nuclei of many kinds of atoms, commonly hydrogen, are tiny magnets. In the Earth's magnetic field they line up to some extent just as you walk around. When you walk past a piece of iron, they'll flop around in different directions. We may think of us as having microscopic compass needles precessing (spinning on their axes like gyroscopes) in an orderly direction. To make an MR image, this tendency of the nuclei to line up in the direction of a magnetic field is manipulated and measured. Since the nuclei from different regions of the body can be made to precess at different frequencies, these frequencies yield signals that are location dependent. Computer images can then be calculated, enhanced, and displayed. (Dawson 2013, 3)

Magnetic resonance imaging, therefore, is—quite literally—a dynamic reconfiguring of the world (Barad 2003). Nuclei, hydrogen magnets, and space and place intra-act with the earth's core while simultaneously intra-acting with computers that calculate, enhance, and display locations and frequencies. Intra-acting phenomena enliven and make visible a body in flux.

Along with MRI scans, the radiological images typically used to diagnosis, treat, and prognosticate about cancer include X-rays, CT scans, PET scans, and ultrasounds. According to Dr. Marco, the PET scan is one of the only radiological imaging techniques characterized as "dynamic" (whereas the rest are considered "static"). Dr. Marco explains that the PET scan allows viewers to see biological activities and processes: "They can also do some metabolic studies—like PET scan is actually a dynamic study because you're looking at metabolic activity of a process occurring in the body and based on its degree of metabolic activity you can ... you're able to establish the likelihood of it [cancer] being malignant or not." Conducting a PET scan involves injecting a small amount of radioactive glucose into the patient's vein and then using a scanner to make colorful and detailed digital pictures of areas inside a body where glucose is taken up and used. Bright colors in an image's final rendering indicate metabolic activity in a patient's tissues. Higher levels of metabolic activity in anatomical areas of concern may suggest the presence of disease. The visualizing techniques of these scans, therefore, render visible a body's otherwise undetectable cellular and metabolic activity. Although they are but snapshots of a freeze-framed moment in time, these images' material methods for production (i.e., radioactive glucose intra-acting with metabolic processes that thereby render bright colors) craft a more dynamic snapshot of bodies' matter, movement, and change over time than X-rays are capable of.

Dr. Thomas indicates that radiological images displayed during tumor board deliberations sometimes allow him "to see whether or not a tumor might be sitting next to a blood vessel, or impairing the patient's breathing by taking up the entire lung." He asserts that such visual displays are important when he considers his patient's overall well-being, not just the management of his patient's cancer. That is, radiological images provide Dr. Thomas with a sense of whether and how a tumor in one part of the body may have a detrimental effect on other parts of the body. Here again, visuals-as-evidence act as maps that provide a rich understanding of how oncologic matter intra-acts with an otherwise healthy body. Visuals help explain why a patient with a particular form of cancer in one part of their body might be experiencing back pain or difficulty walking. Dr. Thomas describes it this way:

> Seeing those images will change minds. Not always, but they can. Sometimes a nodule will light up on a PET scan. That lighting up tells me that maybe this patient might be at risk for a bone fracture if the patient has a bone cancer. If a CT scan shows a mass on the left side of the patient's body, I know I need to pay more attention to if and when this patient has pain in their left side as that might be an indication that the cancer

has spread to other areas. I might not have had an appreciation for that prior to seeing the actual image of that patient's body on the screen.

The evincing power of the radiological image, at least according to Dr. Thomas, is that it allows medical professionals to see disease within the larger context of a patient's whole body. The doctor caring for the patient becomes attuned and attentive to when and how a patient's disease might change and subsequently affect surrounding anatomy.

While X-rays are typically characterized as static black-and-white detections of broken bones, when coupled with other radiological imaging techniques, they make possible a more complex understanding of a body's relationship with matter, movement, and time. Thanks to such visualizations, medical professionals can begin to negotiate the complexities of a body in flux. When coupled with pathological visualization techniques, medical professionals can learn even more about the complexities of a body in flux.

## Pathological Images

In the case of cancer care, attuning evidentially to matter, movement, and time at a cellular level is even more revealing. In an interview with Dr. Marco, I asked him to describe differences between radiological and pathological images in terms of what they argumentatively afford medical professionals.

> Well, look at it this way. It's like you have a sphere. And the disease entity, if you will, is in the center of that sphere. You can approach the disease from different perspectives, and some perspectives use different mediums to see it. Radiology and pathology are both visual disciplines. We both ask: How many different ways can we capture the reality of the patient in terms that we can interpret and render a finding? It's like this microscope here. This microscope here has five objectives: lower power ... all the way up to higher power. Radiology can only go so far. It has limits of assessment and at that point, if you read their reports, they'll say "cannot rule out. . . ." They tend to stay grouped—you know, they'll tell you what general category you're in. With pathology—there's so many ways you can look at things. With the naked eye. You know, patient has a tumor, surgeon takes it out, sets it down, we look at it. We have a fairly straightforward way of assessing it—size, color, consistency, is it solid, cystic, so on and so forth. And then we turn it over to the microscope.

By partnering with a high-powered microscope (see fig. 2.1), Dr. Marco becomes attuned to intra-actions between cancerous cells, tissues, and their

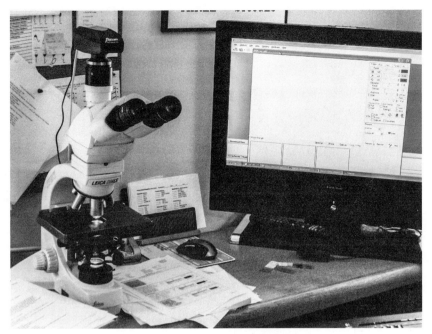

Figure 2.1 Dr. Marco's desk, high-powered microscope

contexts. In other words, the microscope is more than mere instrument or tool. The high-powered microscope is an apparatus that is central to "open-ended and dynamic material-discursive practices, through which specific 'concepts' and 'things' are articulated" (Barad 2007, 334). Apparatuses such as the high-powered microscope are "material configurations (dynamic re-configurings) of the world that play a role in the production of phenomena" (Barad 2007, 335). Microscopes and the vital objects they observe "are specific material performances of the world" (Barad 2007, 335). Through these material performances of the world, pathology images can be used to diagnose cancer, stage cancer (i.e., estimate how advanced a particular cancer is), and predict how bodies might respond to specific medical interventions.

Rendering pathological images requires reliance on a range of material-discursive techniques. Dr. Marco explains that lab technicians place tissue samples taken during a biopsy through a processor overnight so that by the time technicians return to the laboratory in the morning the tissue samples are fully dehydrated. Technicians then place the dehydrated tissue samples in a paraffin wax. Once the wax is cool, technicians place the tissue on an instrument called a microtome. From there, technicians slice a thin, six- to eight-micron section from the now fossilized tissue sample, and they place

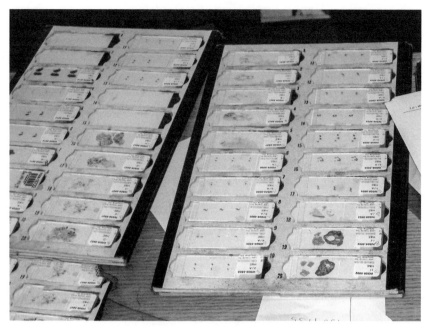

Figure 2.2 Pathology evidences (Dr. Marco's desk)

this section on a glass slide, stain it, add a coverslip to it, and bring it to the pathologist for interpretation. Dr. Marco describes that on any given day he has "maybe five of these trays . . . at about twenty slides on a tray . . . so maybe a hundred slides a day" and that "each case has anywhere from one to twenty-four slides, depending on the complexity of the case." Just in this one pathological technique, and before the official, expert gaze of the pathologist (which is not to suggest other gazes don't precede the pathologist's or that such gazes are any less expert), the evidencing apparatus's material complexity has had its hands in any and all potential findings (see fig. 2.2.). What you see in figure 2.2 is a freeze-framed visual result of the following material intra-actions: radioactive glucose / metabolic processes / tissue samples / change from night to day (required to cure the specimen) / dehydration process / liquid wax / cool air in surrounding environment / microtomes / six-to eight-micron sections / tool used to thinly slice sections / glass / stain / coverslip.[4]

According to Dr. Marco, pathologists sometimes conduct what tumor board participants referred to as a FISH (fluorescent in situ hybridization) study. During FISH studies, pathologists partner with a fluorescent probe that binds to specific places on DNA sequences located within a cancer cell's chromosome. Depending on the makeup of the cancer cell's DNA, the fluorescent binders light up or glow. This technique assumes individual cancer cells have an agency all their own that will manifest in intra-actions with fluorescent binders. Should a visually identifiable intra-action occur, the result is evidentially revealing.

In addition to FISH studies, another method for attuning to cancer's microscopic matter and movement over time is pathological staining. The black-and-white smears on Dr. Marco's slides in figure 2.1 result from a chemical reaction between the unique cellular makeup of the specimen taken from patients' bodies and a particular kind of dye—typically hematoxylin and eosin. Pathologists set the stage for this intra-action during a procedure that Dr. Marco refers to as "an H&E." Interestingly, hematoxylin is a black dye made from compounds that have been extracted from logwood trees. Such trees are native to southern Mexico and northern Central America and played a central role in the creation of fabric dyes. On its own, or when neutral, the dye is a brownish shade. But because hematoxylin is chemically basic, it is attracted to and will bind with acidic compounds. When the dye is attracted to and binds with acidic compounds, it turns a shade of yellow or red, or some combination thereof. When alkaline, hematoxylin turns shades of dark blue and purple. After hematoxylin is added to a tissue sample, laboratory technicians may then deploy a technique called "counterstaining," which involves adding an alcoholic solution called eosin Y. By mobilizing the intra-actional material properties of chemically basic hematoxylin and chemically acidic eosin, technicians visualize cancer cells that render as varying degrees of red, pink, and orange. These colors are the result of an attraction between and binding of acidic eosin and basic proteins.

Patterns in certain cancer cells' shade-based transformations have made staining a suasive method for evidencing disease. In sum, cancer cells' unique chemical makeup finds affinity with the unique chemical makeup of particular dyes. Such a technique hinges on unique and visually detectable intra-actions between different chemical compounds. Resultant images are evidentially revealing. Dr. Marco describes it this way: "Depending on the type of cancer cell, the stain will either be taken up or attracted to certain characteristics of the cancer cell. By observing how colored dye either is or is not taken up by particular parts of the cell, we're able to (a) identify the type of cancer cells they have collected and (b) predict how it may or may not favorably respond to certain kinds of therapies or treatments." Details about how potential cancer cells taken from a patient's body do or do not "take up" dyes are communicated to the surgeon or oncologist caring for the patient through a formal report, phone conversation, or during the tumor board. These details help deliberators decide what kinds of biomedical interventions may or may not be effective in treating a patient's unique cancer. Pathology information can also be generative for deciding whether a patient is eligible to participate in a clinical trial (see chap. 4 for a more in-depth discussion of clinical trials and evidential attunement). Since (at least at the time I conducted this study) it is not a requirement to take a pathology rotation in medical school, pathologists must be present during tumor board deliberations so that they can interpret to deliberators what each image appears to evidence. Not once did I witness challenges from tumor board participants about an image's quality or a pathologist's laboratory method. Not once did details about their backstage staining procedures make an appearance during tumor board deliberations. Even for medical professionals, then, medical images are black-boxed (and necessarily so since tumor board deliberations last only sixty minutes and occur once a week).

In my interview with him, Dr. Thomas indicated that he does not hesitate to make a phone call to the pathologist assigned to his patient's case to request that images be faxed or e-mailed to his office "because they can tell me whether or not the margins are clear." He argues that "when we look at the margins we know whether or not the patient needs to go back in to surgery. We can also know where to go in order to get a clear margin." The phrase "clear margin" is used to signify that, after the tumor has been removed surgically, surrounding tissue left behind is free of one of the millions of cancerous cells the tumor shed during its time in the patient's body. Achieving clear margins is key to providing a patient with a promising prognosis. Here, it seems that in order to anticipate future cellular flux, Dr. Thomas is unafraid to perform the interpretive role typically played by the pathologist. Although Dr. Thomas clarified that his approach for requesting pathological images is not common among his peers, his unique practice demonstrates both the suasive, powerful nature of such visual evidence and the skill required for being able to make inferences about what those images reveal about a body's past, present, and future.

Dr. Thomas goes on to assert that "pathology images are also important because we can tell, by looking at them, how classic looking they are. That is, we can know whether or not the cancer the patient has is a fairly bland cancer or a wild and crazy cancer doing all kinds of crazy things." The pathology image may be the one piece of evidence that can lead to meaningful characterizations of a patient's cancer. While it is important to recognize and account for how medical images are mobilized during deliberative decision making, to truly understand the dynamic and complex nature of how evidence comes to be persuasive, it is also important to note the backstage imaging apparatuses and materialities that are ultimately responsible for attuning to cancer's matter and movement over time.

## ATTUNING VISUALLY TO MOVEMENT, MATTER, AND TIME

Now that readers have a better understanding of the backstage biomedical methods and materials that help make visual evidences persuasive in the first place, the latter half of this chapter reports specific details about the role of medical images during actual patient case presentations. Based on these data, I perform fine-grained analyses of how medical professionals rely on particular evidencing methods for attuning visually to cancer's matter and movement over time.

## Clarice's Case

In patient case presentation seven, deliberation ensued about a forty-eight-year-old female who underwent a vaginal hysterectomy because of fibroids. For the purposes of this analysis, I refer to her as Clarice, although patient names are never used during the tumor board deliberations I observed, nor did I have access to her actual identity. Unlike the next two analyses of patient case presentations, it's necessary for me to provide additional background so that readers can get a sense of the unique complexity of Clarice's case, including how her cancer was detected, how it could be treated, and whether an insurance company would reject her doctors' preferred treatment plan.

During an otherwise routine hysterectomy to remove fibroids, Clarice's surgeon claims to have sensed an irregularity (in his own words, he "just had a bad feeling about it") and decided to send one of her ovaries for a frozen section. A frozen section procedure is when, in the middle of a surgery, the surgeon removes a tissue sample from the area of concern and sends the sample to the pathology laboratory to be analyzed. The advantage of this particular procedure is that the pathologist renders a speedy and somewhat reliable diagnosis while the patient is still on the operating table. If, while Clarice is on the operating table, the pathologist is able to detect the presence or spread of cancer cells, her surgeon can intervene in that moment, rather than having to wait for postoperative results. Here, Clarice's surgeon negotiates with the possibility of ongoing changes in cancer's matter and movement over time by circumventing the wait time required by the typical pathological method for analyzing biopsied tissue. As readers are likely aware, every time a body is opened up during surgery, the patient is exposed to a host of dangers, including infection. This is to say nothing of the risk associated with anesthesia. To try and prevent multiple surgeries, surgeons may order a frozen section of a patient's tissue during surgery. Despite obvious affordances of a rapid biopsy, the slower method (preserving tissue from Clarice's tumor in a paraffin wax and then analyzing it) is the preferred and more reliable technique. Clarice's pathologist notes that he detected no carcinoma in the frozen sample that was analyzed during her surgery. But after the surgery was complete, the pathologist completed the more time-consuming but reliable pathological analysis and detected the presence of endometrial cancer cells.

Remember that originally Clarice was undergoing a rather routine hysterectomy because of fibroids. Without her surgeon's felt sense that something else was at work, Clarice's cancer may have gone undetected for some time. This was, therefore, an incidental finding of cancer. One reason medical professionals brought Clarice's case to the attention of the tumor board is because there is not a clear, standard protocol for how to proceed when cancer is found incidentally (see chap. 4 for a more in-depth exploration of medical standards and clinical practice guidelines or protocols). The other indeterminacy motivating the need for expert deliberation in Clarice's case was a question about the cancer's stage. Medical professionals' decisions about how to stage Clarice's endometrial cancer predict how aggressively it could (or should) be treated. In an attempt to resolve these uncertainties, medical professionals deliberated about whether Clarice should undergo a controversial procedure called a pelvic lymphadenectomy. A pelvic lymphadenectomy is an aggressive, nonstandard procedure in which lymph nodes are removed from a patient's pelvis and sent to a pathologist for gross and microscopic analysis. Such a procedure, while nonstandard and controversial, would help resolve the indeterminacies described above. However, because this procedure is costly, and because the detection of Clarice's cancer was incidental, deliberators agreed that most insurance companies would not approve this particular intervention.

Now that readers have a sense of the uncertainties that motivated Clarice's oncologist to bring her case to the attention of the tumor board, what follows is a deliberative trace of all references made, from start to finish, in the order they were made during Clarice's case presentation. (Note: the patient case presentation started at 12:11 because it was the second case presented that day and the first case only lasted twelve minutes and eleven seconds.) I was a lone researcher during this meeting, so keeping track of references and relevant details while also watching the passage of time was difficult (see table 2.3); specific times indicated in the far left column, therefore, are approximate. Table 2.3 provides a fairly linear description of the deliberative process during Clarice's case. Tumor board deliberators' specific kinds of references are noted in the middle column while details pertaining to those references

**Table 2.3 Clarice: A Deliberative Trace**

| Time (min:sec) | Kind of Reference | Specific Details |
|---|---|---|
| 12:11— START | Patient's background information | Surgeon describes: this patient is a 68-year-old female who presented with postmenopausal bleeding. Describes patient's risk factors and the fact that she had been on estrogen replacement for osteoporosis (prescribed by her gynecologist, not present). |
| | Question from audience | "Why is the patient on estrogen for bone loss?" Debate ensues about the controversial nature of prescribing the patient estrogen replacement for bone loss. |
| 13:12 | Patient's background information | Surgeon describes that the patient had undergone a vaginal hysterectomy and right salpingo-oophorectomy (removal of fallopian tubes and ovaries) because her gynecologist had diagnosed her with an "enlarged fibroid uterus." |
| | Question from audience | "Why did the patient undergo a vaginal hysterectomy as opposed to an abdominal hysterectomy?" Debate ensues about why patients choose a vaginal over abdominal hysterectomy and concludes with an understanding that recovery time is important to patients. |
| 14:17 | Patient's background information | Surgeon describes that during the vaginal hysterectomy, the surgeon was not able to remove the left ovary and became suspicious that perhaps more was going on than just fibroids. What the surgeon did remove, however, was sent immediately to pathology for a frozen section. |
| 15:05 | Pathological information (oral reference, no visual) | Surgeon describes that "no noted carcinoma" was the verdict of the pathologist's frozen section. |
| 15:19 | Lights dim; images projected. | ... |
| 15:20 | Radiological information (oral + visual) | Radiologist displays four different images from an ultrasound of the patient's pelvis. |

**Table 2.3 Continued**

| Time (min:sec) | Kind of Reference | Specific Details |
|---|---|---|
| 17:29 | Pathological information (oral + visual) | Pathologist displays an image of a "section of" the tissue from the endometrial biopsy. |
| 17:36 | Pathological information (oral + visual) | Pathologist displays image of a section of hysterectomy specimen and notes measurements and "other problems." |
| 17:45 | Pathological information (oral + visual) and typical practice | Pathologist displays image and describes that "our policy" is usually to open the specimen and evaluate the depth of invasion. |
| 17:55 | Pathological information (oral + visual) | Pathologist displays image and describes that it "appears to be noninvasive to my eye." |
| 18:20 | Pathological information (oral + visual) | Pathologist displays an image and describes that only one of 13 sections contained more than "1 mm of invasion." Therefore, margins are clear. |
| 19:25 | Pathological information (oral + visual) | Pathologist displays an image and describes that the tumor occurs on the posterior wall of the uterus and measures 2.5 cm in greatest diameter. |
| 20:00 | Pathological information (oral + visual) | Pathologist displays an image and describes how in this image, seen at "higher power," you can see how the margins are uninvolved by invasive carcinoma and no venous/lymphatic invasion exists. |
| 20:30 | Pathological information (oral + visual) | Pathologist displays an image, describes how this is an example of squamous cell metastases, and declares that this is not an uncommon finding. |
| 20:39 | Standards of care | Debate ensues about how far her cancer has progressed. Tumor board chairperson describes that, based on the imaging, surgically her cancer is a grade 1 of 3. |
| 21:05 | Standards of care | Debate ensues about how best to treat the patient with this cancer grade. Tumor board chairperson describes that her options are (a) surveillance/normal exams or (b) complete her staging, which includes a series of tests and scans. If they're all negative, she undergoes no further treatment. |

**Table 2.3 Continued**

| Time (min:sec) | Kind of Reference | Specific Details |
|---|---|---|
| 21:50 | Question from audience regarding standard of care | "How do we treat an incidental finding of cancer?" Debate ensues about the controversy surrounding whether or not patients like this should undergo a "pelvic lymphadenectomy." |
| 22:30 | Standards of care and pathological information | Tumor board chairperson describes that it's a part of surgical staging but is still controversial; we need to consider additional operative and post-op risks and benefits while also looking at the pathology. |
| 23:05 | Studies and statistics | Oncologist references an article in which 200 patients are a part of a retrospective study and then discusses the statistics involved in this procedure. |
| 23:50 | Studies and statistics | Surgeon is aware of article and the percentages but worries about understaging and undertreating patients. Debate ensues about this article. |
| 26:18— END | | |

are noted in the far right column. The meeting's chronological progression can be followed from top to bottom.

During Clarice's case presentation, the surgeon expresses concern about whether he removed enough tissue to get a "clear margin." Here, the surgeon is referring explicitly to the unpredictability of cancer's movement over time. He is concerned about safely removing just enough of the surrounding tissue so that minimally invasive cancer cells—cells that are not detectable to the surgeon's naked eye—are not left behind to spread after the surgery is over. Surgeons must make these decisions while in the middle of a procedure and while remaining mindful of how tumors sometimes press against vital organs, blood vessels, and bones. Despite standards of care documents that attempt to create uniform guidelines as to how much of the surrounding tissue should be excised, uncertainty about how much tissue to remove is persistent. Saunders (2010) describes this tension best: "Findings too small to characterize are not below the threshold of the significant—but are unquantifiably ambiguous" (19). Grappling with unquantifiable ambiguity, medical professionals often rely on imaging as evidence for determining how clear the margins are. Medical images lessen the ambiguity but never fully erase it.

In Clarice's case, only one of thirteen sections show a less than one-millimeter invasion of tumor cells. Such a result is evidence in support of a fairly good prognosis for Clarice. However, as I described earlier, these evidences are backed by methods that hinge on mere slices of slices of slices of a specimen. So while medical imaging helps pathologists diagnose and prognosticate about a patient's cancer, medical images' argumentative affordances must be traced back not only to the surgeon's in situ decision making about where to locate his or her device when excising tissue, but also to backstage materials and techniques that help coconstruct the final, rendered medical image now on display in the front of the room.

Exploring the surgeon's skillful in situ decision making while Clarice was on the operating table is beyond the scope of this chapter, but it is tempting to characterize such skill as another form of backstage evidential practice akin to what Sauer (2003) and Haas and Witte (2001) might call embodied knowledge. Embodied knowledge alone is not enough, however. The surgeon partners with things—materials and techniques—as a way to warrant evidential claims. In Clarice's case, two imaging methods are deployed: (1) pathological analysis of a frozen section and (2) an ultrasound. Images from these methods attune the surgeon and tumor board deliberators to the spread of cancer cells in areas surrounding the primary tumor. Seeing evidence of spread provides medical deliberators with the information required to stage Clarice's cancer.[5]

According to the pathologist working on Clarice's case, on interpretation, visual displays indicate (a) the presence, (b) the type, and (c) the stage of the cancer. Taken together, these three crucial pieces of bioinformation about cancer's matter and movement over time are necessary when making decisions about how a patient can (or should) be treated. Medical images of Clarice's cancer not only provide evidence for the microscopic presence of cancer—which was virtually undetectable at under one millimeter—but also provide evidence that medical professionals then use to name the cancer and determine how far it has progressed.

### Sadie's Case

In another patient case presentation, a seventy-seven-year-old female (hereafter, "Sadie") with a medical history that includes resected colon cancer and several other life-threatening health conditions (referred to as "comorbidities")—that is, gout, arthritis, mild renal failure, long-term steroid use—is presented to the tumor board. Sadie's case is complex because she is experiencing excruciating pain from spinal cord compression, which is a symptom of colon cancer after it has progressed. After Sadie's oncologist presents her patient's age, biological sex, medical history, family history, and "social history" (Sadie was once a pack-a-day smoker who quit eight years ago), the radiologist presents his findings.

The radiologist gestures toward and describes how a bright red hotspot on the PET scan displayed on a screen in the front of the room shows "abnormal activity in the left upper cervical posterior paraspinal tumor, and the destruction of two vertebrae." He suggests the possibility of metastatic colon carcinoma. Additional details from imaging results are presented, including results from an abdominal/pelvic CT scan; separate CT scans of the chest, pelvis, and lumbar spine; a bone scan; an MRI of the cervical spine; and a PET scan. While images from the CT scan are presented to the tumor board, the radiologist affixes tiny red arrows on the actual slide to draw deliberators' attention to small nodules hiding out in the right lower lobe of Sadie's lungs. The radiologist then displays the most recent CT scan alongside a CT scan that had been performed several months earlier. Side by side, these two scans allow tumor board participants to see, by way of comparison, that since Sadie's last exam the right lower lobe mass had grown and "become lobulated, in addition to two smaller nodules present." Radiological images, in Sadie's case, visually attune deliberators to changes in cancer's matter and movement over time.

After the radiologist presents and describes his visual findings, the pathologist presents a series of images rendered in his laboratory. The pathologist explains that each of the images displayed on-screen indicate that Sadie's cancer cells are "invasive" (meaning they have spread to other parts of her body, beyond the immediate tissue where the tumor was originally located). Moreover, Sadie's cancer cells are "moderately to poorly differentiated" (meaning Sadie's tumor cells are changing and look quite unlike healthy cells—evidence that supports a poor prognosis). Deliberation ensues about how to manage Sadie's pain since, given her age and other comorbidities, Sadie is not a good candidate for aggressive cancer treatment.

In Sadie's case, then, red hotspots, comparative CT scans, and microscopic renderings of the nature of her cancer cells attune deliberators to the existence, type, and seriousness of disease. With these data, medical professionals decide that the disease was detected well after the cancer had first arrived on scene, thereby lessening the chances that any operation, chemotherapy, or radiation treatment will do more good than harm. Images of Sadie's cancer help prepare oncologists to make decisions about palliative care rather than aggressive and invasive treatments that stand to lessen Sadie's quality of life without much of a chance for actual improvement in her oncologic condition.

## Monika's Case

As was the case for both Clarice and Sadie, methods for visually attuning to cancer assist medical professionals as they evidence disease and make decisions about whether the patient is a candidate for specific treatments and interventions. Monika, a fifty-four-year-old female patient, endured a mastectomy of her right breast eight years prior to this tumor board meeting and was subsequently treated with Tamoxifen for five years. The complexity in Monika's case is attributable to what occurred during a routine examination: Monika's oncologist discovered a small, palpable nodule over her surgical scar. Other than this tiny lump, Monika had no complaints or symptoms. After her oncologist presents Monika's background information—medical history, a description of all previously performed surgical procedures, the fact that Monika's father died of lymphoma, and that Monika quit smoking thirty years ago—the radiologist and pathologist present their images.

The lights are dimmed and a black-and-white image of a skeleton's chest is displayed, on which tumor board participants can see a rather large, red hotspot near the skeleton's left side. The radiologist gestures toward the red hotspot, saying, "This is the area of palpable concern." He then presents results from PET and CT scans that indicate "no evidence of metastatic disease or hypermetabolic activity in the axillary lymph nodes." He explains, though, that the PET scan, as evidenced by the red hotspot on the screen, shows somewhat increased metabolic activity in the chest wall nodule. The radiologist hypothesizes, therefore, that this may be (*a*) evidence of recurrent carcinoma, (*b*) merely postoperative granulation tissue (i.e., scarring from her previous surgery), or (*c*) both. Uncertainty surrounding which of these possibilities is most probable intensifies the complexity of Monika's case.

Next, the pathologist reports that Monika's surgeon removed the mastectomy scar and surrounding tissue and sent the tissue sample to the pathology laboratory. The tissue underwent the usual pathologic protocol, including a hematoxylin and eosin stain, and was viewed under a high-powered microscope. This view provides evidence of the "scattered" nature of the cells. Moreover, their "scattered, buckshot appearance, which can be easily missed at lower power," provides evidence that these cells had, in fact, "infiltrated the lobular." The pathologist also describes that the nuclei of Monika's tumor cells are "positive" (for cancer) and reports that after adding a blue-gray counterstain to the cells and viewing them under a microscope set to lower power, she was able to see that cells had spread to what was referred to as a "subcutaneous area." The pathologist hypothesizes that this spread of cells is what is responsible for the palpable nodule beneath Monika's surgery scar. She provides additional detail about Monika's cancer cells by describing how, at the time of observation, they were lined up in a row, forming a cancer-filled barrier in a pattern he referred to as "Indian filing." (Despite the obvious cultural insensitivity, this term is, in fact, an actual term used by some pathologists and other medical professionals.)

After pathological images from Monika's tumor are displayed and described, deliberation ensues about which treatments will be most effective. Monika's oncologist explains that there is "no good data" about what to do in cases like Monika's. A reference is made to the FISH study that the pathologist performed earlier, which indicates that Monika's tumor tested positively for HER-2/neu (a protein that is detected in cases of particularly aggressive cancer). Monika's positive result for this protein makes her an eligible candidate for Herceptin treatment, should she agree to this more aggressive approach. Tumor board deliberators agree that this treatment option should be presented to Monika and her care network as one possibility for future action.

In each of the cases described above, medical images evince and attune deliberators to cancer's matter and movement over time. Radiologists' and pathologists' verbal descriptions are paired with visual displays of body data, and taken together they make up the evidence medical professionals use to name cancer, leverage claims about its nature, and predict its future behavior. The case presentations for Clarice, Sadie, and Monika provide a backstage look at how materials (e.g., stains, slides, and scopes) make matter mean during real-time deliberations. Table 2.4 maps the relationship between backstage methods and materials, how those methods and materials attune deliberators to cancer's matter and movement, and how those attunements result in certain argumentative affordances.

In sum, the relationship between backstage methods and materials, evidential attunements, and argumentative affordances might best be summarized in the following ways.

1. By placing images alongside one another that have been rendered at different chronological times (but from the same body), deliberators attune to change over time. Here, deliberators are able to more readily see whether a cancer treatment has worked or if a tumor has grown or reduced in size, and they can thereby make evidence-based decisions about possible treatment options.
2. By using dyes to highlight (quite literally through bright red hotspots) metabolic activity, deliberators attune to chemical reactions

## Table 2.4 Methods for Visual Attunements and Evidences

| Method | Attunements | Evidence |
|---|---|---|
| Rendering present an image of one object of study alongside a later image of the same object of study | Attuning to change over time | Evidence about whether a cancer treatment has worked<br><br>Evidence about whether a tumor has grown or shrunk |
| Rendering present black and white behind red hotspot | Attuning to metabolic processes | Evidence about the cancer's malignancy |
| Rendering present dark red on top of blue-gray | Attuning to hormone positivity or negativity | Evidence about the patient's eligibility for particular treatments |
| Rendering present a dark shadow (i.e., tumor) next to or near other vital organs, tissues, or bones | Attuning to the effect a tumor has on other bodily parts and processes | Evidence about how other anatomical structures are threatened and how the patient's quality of life may be affected by the cancer |
| Rendering present cells that are lined up in a row | Attuning to "Indian filing" | Evidence about the cancer's invasiveness and how it might respond to treatment |
| Rendering present through high-powered and low-powered views | Attuning to cancer cells' differentiation | Evidence about the cancer's stage |
| | Attuning to how actively the cells are dividing | Evidence about the cancer's stage |
| | Attuning to how big the nuclei are | Evidence about the cancer's malignancy (if nuclei are pleomorphic), or about it being benign (nuclei are small and regular) |
| | Attuning to whether the margins are clear | Evidence about the cancer's invasiveness and whether returning to surgery is warranted |

characteristic of cellular growth and activity. Malignant (versus benign) cancers demonstrate higher levels of metabolic activity. Seeing the presence (or not) of metabolic activity allows for evidence-based debates to ensue regarding possible treatment options. If metabolic activity is not present, for example, it's possible a surgical or pharmaceutical intervention would be unnecessary.

3. By using stains that are (or are not) taken up, depending on the material and hormonal makeup of the cancer cell, deliberators attune to cancer cells' hormone positivity or negativity. As we saw with Monika's cancer, some tumors (in particular, breast cancers) are characterized as either "hormone positive" or "hormone negative"; depending on that characterization, tumor cells will respond more or less readily to specific treatments. In the next chapter, for instance, I describe the case of a breast cancer drug called Avastin, which is a treatment that was once used in advanced stage, hormone-positive breast cancers. Based on resultant colors rendered in the pathology laboratory, deliberators embark on evidence-based discussions about the patient's eligibility for certain treatments, such as Avastin, Herceptin, or some combination thereof.

4. By using a concentrated beam of electrons that intra-acts differently with different parts of a body, deliberators attune to a tumor's spatial relationship with organs, tissues, and bones of critical import. The fact that the soft tissues of a body cannot absorb an X-ray's beams makes it possible for radiologists to detect material densities and thereby diagnose the presence of masses or lesions. Locating cancer's material conditions and how they intra-act with vital organs, tissues, or bones attunes deliberators to why a patient might have difficulty eating, sleeping, or walking. Having this visual information on hand prepares deliberators to make evidence-based decisions about how to mitigate pain and improve a patient's quality of life.

5. By using the high- and low-power settings on a microscope, deliberators attune to the degree to which cancer cells have infiltrated or invaded certain parts of their patient's body. If, as we saw in Monika's case, cancer cells are lined up in a row, forming a kind of defense barrier, this affects a patient's options for treatment. Similarly, microscopic views either through high or low power attune deliberators to cellular differentiation, how actively they are dividing, how large the nuclei are, and whether the area surrounding a tumor (i.e., margins) is free from cancer cells. Having this visual information

on hand is of critical importance for making evidence-based decisions about care options.

Each of the above evidential attunements enable evidence-based deliberation and decision making about patients' treatment options, in particular whether surgery to remove a tumor and surrounding regions (also known as "getting clear margins") might be beneficial. Backstage biomedical visualization methods enact or perform cancer. Because of what they reveal when cancer is viewed from close or from far away, evidencing bodies visually helps deliberators negotiate medical uncertainty.

### ATTUNING KAIROTICALLY TO BODIES IN FLUX

Had I more skill, I would attempt to map matter, movement, and time onto a three-dimensional space to illustrate how medical professionals attune themselves to bodies in flux. That illustration would demonstrate a host of well-orchestrated intra-acting collisions and partnerships that result in observable phenomena: cancer cells collide with the effects of refrigeration; the surgeon's hand partners with a scalpel, then partners with the dynamics of a patient's body multiple (Mol 2002); glass slides collide with magnetic force; patients' time collides with cancer's time. The vectors of intra-action are innumerable.

In her description of how atherosclerosis is performed or "enacted," Mol (2002) notes that "formaldehyde, staining fluids, knives, slides, microscopes" (54) play a central role. She proposes a praxiographic understanding of disease, which posits that local matters and practices determine what is. For Mol, a praxiographic or practice-based approach is a markedly different approach to disease and care than an epistemological approach. The proposed three-dimensional map I describe above would illustrate how "objects-in-practice have complex relations" (Mol 2002, 149). Objects described in Mol's "Hospital Z" as well as the medical images described above "do not so much cohere as assemble" (150). Radioactive glucose, dyes derived from trees, paraffin wax, processors, and dozens of other assembling agents participate in performing that which we come to call cancer.

Results from analyses above demonstrate that medical images are more than representations that signify, represent, or are "read" in a literary sense (in the manner suggested by Kress and van Leeuwen 2006). They *do* more than they *display*. Indeed, it is possible to theorize visualizations of disease in terms of reading and writing, as Saunders (2010) posits in *CT Suite: The Work of Diagnosis in the Age of Noninvasive Cutting*. But analyses I present here suggest that, when we give objects their due (Marback 2008), visualizations of disease are local performances of a cellular and molecular world that, despite their explanatory power in that moment, are constrained by the inevitability of change over time yet to be visualized.

Medical professionals negotiate with the inevitability of change over time by evidencing bodies through what Haraway (1991) might refer to as a series of "visualizing tricks and powers of modern sciences and technologies" (188–90). Echoing Haraway, Keller (2009) challenges the romantic assumption that looking and touching in science are mutually exclusive practices. In fact, Keller argues that by looking, or as a result of our biological gaze, we intervene, manipulate, and alter.[6] To challenge assumptions about scientific objectivity, both Haraway (1991) and Keller (2009) focus almost exclusively on how humans manipulate, intervene, and alter scientific materials. Drawing on Niels Bohr, Keller (2009) argues that, "if we have learned anything from physics at all, it is of the impossibility, even in the physical domain, of looking without touching: the very light we shine disturbs the object at which we gaze" (117). Elkins (1996) similarly asserts that even "weightless looking" ("typing ... glancing at my hands and up at the screen, looking over at my empty coffee cup") is "directed" (21). Such an assertion—that all looking is, in fact, directed—is not necessarily new, particularly among scholars who study visualization in medicine (see Cartright 1995; Dumit 2004; Fountain 2014; Ihde 2002; Prentice 2012; Segal 2005; Stafford 1993; van Dijck 2005). And yet, as Ihde (2002) insists, "In so far as I use a technology, I am also used by a technology" (137). Visual evidence, therefore, is a coconstructive performance. Just as Lynch (2006) concluded in his analysis of scientific visual displays of animals' bodies: "Data were neither wholly out there in the animals' anatomy, nor wholly constructed out of thin air" (215). Data are coconstructed performances.

Understanding visual rhetorics in medicine as coconstructed performances means we must reconsider long-held assertions about how humans construct bodies (see Klaver 2009, e.g.). While it is true that "the objects to which (medical) images refer are always mediated by the very instruments and methods used to depict them" (Pasveer 2006, 43; see also Cohen and Meskin 2004; Kulvicki 2010), we must remain mindful that such accounts rely heavily on human exceptionalism. That is, the expert human gaze exerts a kind of epistemological hegemony on the thing as of yet unknown. Such accounts reinforce the very subject-object relationships that feminist thinkers like Haraway have sought to dissolve.

In this chapter, I have strived neither to undermine human expertise in the scientific laboratory nor to neglect the mediational means by which visual evidences are constructed. Rather, I have demonstrated that matter, movement, and time collide in local spaces and places to perform one momentary act of oncological being in a lengthy theatrical production (of which we have only a partial perspective). Theorizing medical visualizations in this way allows us to account more holistically for evidencing as a verb, a practice, or performance—not necessarily a static and perfect object rendered expertly in a laboratory. Intra-actions between humans, nonhumans, space, matter, and time *evince*. Medical images embody one performance of disease at a specific moment in time. That is what they *do*. Our part in cancer's choreography is to go on improvising and negotiating with the materiality of disease through a series of intra-actions that bear up and make possible that which we come to know.

Negotiating constant change over time—cellular or otherwise—requires a kind of rhetorical dwelling. Dwelling, according to Rickert (2013), is "how people come together . . . in the continual making of a place; at that same time, that place is interwoven into the way they have come to be as they are" (xiii). Dwelling, therefore, requires we forgo the temptation to position the human and all our gazing expertise on the front lines of managing cancer's indeterminacy. Dwelling requires we acknowledge the hubris involved in declaring the human gaze as that which is wholly responsible for seeing and thereby knowing a body. Indeed, like Scribner's kaleidoscope, which I reference in this chapter's epigraph, the tools we use shape both what is seen and the very seeable object, itself. But this is not the whole story. How and what we see is a never-ending negotiation with matter, movement, and time.

As the rate of cancer deaths rises despite advances in imaging technologies, it is tempting to either deploy cancer-fighting narratives that position a body as a rogue actor in a sea of invasion or to claim that "our inner bodies are stubbornly incommunicative" (Belling 2010, 232).[7] I part ways with such narratives—narratives that argue that "it is the patient who must interpolate the cancer . . . through the intentional (and usually collaborative and medical) production of meaning we call diagnosis" (Belling 2010, 232; see also Leander [2008] and Little et al.'s [1998] notion of "liminality"). In this chapter, I demonstrate that, in fact, our bodies are quite communicative. Rather than continue to characterize bodies as stubbornly incommunicative or declare war against them, we must make peace with the fact that seeing is and always will be both a situated and partial practice.

Bodies in flux outpace the human gaze. To assume or act otherwise is a political act fraught with competing values. That is, mobilizing the human gaze as a way to make claims about the beginnings and end of cellular life is usually a means to some political, social, or economic end (e.g., proclama-

*Chapter 2*

tions about fetal personhood). To deploy discursive characterizations of cancer cells as "mutant," "invasive," "renegade," and having a kind of "agenda" is to promulgate militaristic paradigms that vilify bodies. Such metaphorical warspeak, in turn, obligates patients and medical professionals to "fight," "defend," and "defeat" the cancerous enemy inside. Garrison (2007) deftly argues that in the case of the so-called war against breast cancer we need to be better aware of "not only the historical, cultural and social conditions giving rise to this metaphor, but also the potentially negative consequences of drafting women, and those who love them, into a sustained conflict against the self" (n.p.). I echo Garrison's (2007) argument and hope that how we narrate cancer might better account for how disease involves corporeal-environmental intra-actions. Space matters. Movement matters. Time matters. A focus on fighting and defeating our turncoat bodies (especially at the level of the gene, as discussed in chap. 5) distances us from attending to the very environmental conditions that contribute to cancer-causing agents in the first place.[8] Rather than propagating vapid anthropocentric narratives of fighting or battling against bodies, to dwell rhetorically with disease requires that we address the political, economic, environmental, and corporeal vectors of intra-action that affect local, global, and cellular bodies' movement and matter over time.[9]

In a previous report of this study, I used Perelman and Olbrechts-Tyteca's (1969) construct, presence, to explain how the visual display of evidence during tumor board deliberations facilitated a move from uncertainty into certitude about possibilities for future action. Specifically, "the very fact of selecting certain elements and presenting them to the audience, their importance and pertinency to the discussion are implied. Indeed, such a choice endows these elements with a presence, which is an essential factor in argumentation and one that is far too much neglected in rationalistic conceptions of reasoning" (Perelman 1982, 116). Perelman argues that "presence acts directly upon our sensibility" and "the presentation of an object ... can effectively move the audience or the jury" (35). I see now, however, that presence fails to account for the complexity of the materials and methods by which biological chaos assembles well prior to the deliberative moment. Ignorant of the role of nonhuman actors and material feminist scholarship, in general, I placed human expertise at the center of biomedical practice. Akin to others who attend to how medical images are rhetorical (e.g., Cartwright 1995; Dumit 2004; van Dijck 2005), I failed to explicate associations between backstage material-discursive practices and human-nonhuman actors involved in imaging medical evidence. That is, I failed to account for presences that precede methods for manipulating laboratory matter. Recall Rickert's (2013) admonishment: "Rhetoric cannot be reduced to the intent—deliberate or posited—to persuade, for we have to include the larger background, including our activity against which the particular assemblage of elements comes to be seen as suasive" (160). By shifting slightly my object of analysis from the deliberative moment (the tumor board) onto predeliberative methods for attuning to a body in constant flux, a world of actors, actants, and activities suddenly became available to me as a researcher.

Tissue culture theorists have for some time attended to that which precedes methods of laboratory manipulation. They suggest that cells have an agency or life of their own (see, e.g., Landecker 2002, 2004). Noting the agentic capacity of cells, Jayna Brown (2015) posits that Henrietta Lacks's "HeLa" cells were "the first to survive 'immortality' outside the body" (321). Not only does a materialist-rhetorical approach to medical images force us to acknowledge cancer cells' agency, but it also forces us to destabilize normative narratives of life, death, and humanity in general. As Jayna Brown (2015) argues: "Situating ourselves at the cellular level shows us that our supposedly discrete bodies are actually complex ecosystems of cells, bacteria, and other organisms, which challenges our notion of individuality and sovereignty" (326). The challenge now, at least from ethical, medical, and rhetorical standpoints, is to resist the impulse to colonize cellular and molecular life and to learn, instead, how to dwell with and among their multiplicity.[10]

I posit that dwelling with a rapidly changing assemblage of not-quite-human objects—cancer cells and other organic and inorganic (e.g., environmental pollution) materials—is more a matter of *kairos* than presence. Amid the collision of matter, movement, and time, medical professionals attune kairotically to onco-corporeal flux. Here I don't necessarily mean *kairos* in the sense of proper timing and good measure. As Hawhee (2002), Miller (1994), and Scott (2006) demonstrate, *kairos* as a rhetorical construct can be and is richer than proper timing and good measure. Recall Eskin's (2002) reminder that *kairos* was actually a practical guide for Hippocrates. Key to Hippocrates's understanding of *kairos* was that it was "not just about time" (Eskin 2002, 105) but about "changing environments" (98), "questions of degree" (100), and "situational context" (111). Similarly, Rickert's (2013) definition for *kairos* requires a sense of "material emplacement and unfolding" rather than "timeliness or decorum" (76). In fact, *kairos* has always located its etymological and practical roots in sensitivity to body and place. In his historically rich outline of how *kairos* emerged as a construct, Rickert (2013) locates its origins in Homer's reference to a specific point on the body where an "arrow finds its mark" (77); later, *kairos* is associated with the Romans' *tempus*, from which we get our word for "temple," or "weak and easily penetrable points on the skull" (78). Rickert (2013) argues that *kairos* takes on a sense of "achievement of workable or probable truths in situations lacking certainty" (81) and that it both "includes and transcends human doing" (83). Indeed, a theory of *kairos* that is limited to "temporal, opportunistic, and propitiatory dimensions" (Rickert 2013, 77) has little explanatory power in circumstances where matter, movement, and time overlap in unpredictable if not indeterminate ways. *Kairos*—unlike Perelmanian presence—accounts for ever-changing material localities of being.

Dwelling kairotically is a rhetorical skill required for attuning to spatial and temporal contingencies of constantly changing phenomena. One may liken this skill to that which I alluded earlier regarding Chinese medical practice: "Wang er zhi ... was thus to know things before they had taken form, to grasp 'what is there and yet not there'" (Kuriyama 1999, 179). Rather than place agential emphasis on the eye of the beholder, however, the gazer is but one participant in an assemblage that performs the world. That is, corporeal and cancer objects are always already present; cancer cells do exist even if we cannot yet see them. But the *evidenced* object emerges through a series of material, spatial, and temporal performances. Apparatuses and agencies collide in a local space and moment in time; these apparatuses and agencies go on doing what they do long after the observer finishes doing what they do. In cancer care, we witness, perhaps more readily than in any other context, how discursive decisions as means for managing medical uncertainty are fallible. Cancer care requires dwelling kairotically with and among an assemblage of changing and colliding matter, movement, and time.

In the spirit of multiple ontologies, therefore, it stands to reason that there might be other meaningful ways of imaging and attuning kairotically to cancer. Perhaps attuning kairotically to cancer is possible not just through assemblages of stains, slides, and scopes but also through assemblages of artistic materials, textures, and human experience. By way of example, as I write this, a guest artist at the David Geffen School of Medicine at the University of California, Los Angeles, is teaching medical students how to transform human scars and other local and lived materialities into art. In so doing, this doctor-artist provides "future doctors with a more tangible understanding of living with certain afflictions" (Frank 2015, n.p.). Such an approach to evincing cancer is one way to negotiate with a body in flux or to dwell with disease.

How else might it look to be attuned kairotically to material (and cellular) localities of being? To answer this, allow me to conclude with the following.

In her study of technical documentation in hazardous environments, Sauer's (2003) miners attune kairotically to an intriguingly similar hazardous and unpredictable environment: the coal mine. Sauer makes a persuasive case for acknowledging and documenting how coal miners deploy "pit sense" as a warrant for the decisions they make amid risky situations. Pit sense, a form of "embodied sensory knowledge" (182), consists of "physical sensations felt or perceived in highly specific local environments" (182). As an important first step in challenging the official and fixed authority of scientific knowledge, Sauer's pit sense accounts for how coal miners are, in a way, attuned to and with their material environment. Although she never actually uses attunement or *kairos* as explanatory constructs, her study demonstrates that coal miners' embodied sensory knowledge to matter, movement, and time saves lives. So while it may be said that Sauer, akin to constructivist theorists described above, positions agency in the driver's seat of the human (specifically, the human body as a mediator of risk) and characterizes the material world as mere environment, she at least accounts for (1) how the unique material conditions of nonhuman and not-quite-human environments affect human (well)being and (2) the fraught way in which we try to communicate those effects. For Sauer, the "profound uncertainty" of hazardous environments challenge "conventions of technical writing" and force us into "rethinking the fundamental assumptions that guide rhetorical practice" (124). Sauer's work demonstrates how material-discursive attunements have implications not only for those who are in the trenches, doing work in risky environments, but also for technical communicators, rhetoricians, public policy makers, and public health professionals, in general.

Moving (perhaps clumsily) from the mining pit to the corporeal core of oncological disease, I posit that bodily tissues themselves make up hazardous and unpredictable environments.[11] Even as living matter is disembodied and redistributed in the laboratory, and in spite of biomedicine's attempts at diagnostically narrating its genesis and prognosticating its end, "the cell is ... a central actor in today's biomedical, biological, and biotechnical settings" (Landecker 2007, 4).[12] The capacity to dwell amid cellularly hazardous and unpredictable environments relies on *kairos* as a rhetorical skill.

Enlivening *kairos* as an explanatory construct for how medical professionals and patients might attempt to make peace with or negotiate cancer's indeterminacy, this chapter describes the "vectors of material and discursive force" (Rickert 2013, 90) involved in attuning to bodies in flux. By shifting from seeing the human (scientists, doctor, patient) as the prime mover in cancer care toward understanding the complexity of cancer care's assemblages and attunements, *kairos* is reimagined as more than the opportunistic leveraging of time toward some suasive end. Dwelling *kairotically* is a rhetorical skill required for navigating medical uncertainty—a skill made possible because of its capacity to account for matter, movement, and time as suasive contributors to decision making. Dwelling *kairotically* is a rhetorical skill required for care.

# 3. ASSESSING EVIDENCE

*Banal as a winter day or the color of the ceiling,*
*survival statistics offer a smidgeon of information,*
*but not much to cuddle with. How could something be at once*
*so transparent* (you will live or die*) and so pig-headedly*
*confusing* (will you live or die*)?*
S. Lochlann Jain, *Malignant: How Cancer Becomes Us*

Crystal Hanna, a thirty-six-year-old woman who was diagnosed with breast cancer in October 2008 was invited to testify at the Food and Drug Administration's (FDA) Avastin hearing in Silver Spring, Maryland, on June 28, 2011. In her testimony, Crystal described details about her disease experience: shortly after completing a half marathon in her hometown, she was diagnosed with breast cancer and subsequently underwent surgery and six months of chemotherapy followed by seven weeks of daily radiation. After a brief period of remission, her cancer returned two years later. And this time there were multiple tumors in her liver and bones. Crystal's doctors prescribed Avastin, which at that time had been granted accelerated approval for the treatment of end-stage breast cancer.[1] Crystal's primary audience — members of the FDA — understood that accelerated approval status is granted if a clinical benefit can be demonstrated. Herein lies the rub.[2]

The FDA defines a clinical benefit as a "positive therapeutic effect that is clinically meaningful in the context of a given disease" (U.S. FDA 2014, n.p.). In an accelerated approval situation there is pressing, unmet clinical need — usually an illness with no known cure — wherein patients like Crystal have limited, if any, treatment options at their disposal. Because data from clinical trials required for full approval might not become available until well after a disease advances irreversibly, the FDA relies on what are called surrogate endpoints as predictors for a drug's therapeutic potential. According to the FDA, a surrogate endpoint is a "laboratory measurement, radiographic image, physical sign or other measure that is thought to predict clinical benefit, but is not itself a measure of clinical benefit" (2014, n.p.). As is also the case in studies required for full FDA approval, clinical trials that demonstrate a drug's effect on a surrogate endpoint must be adequate and controlled. After having been granted accelerated approval in 2008, Genentech (the drug company that developed Avastin) was required to conduct randomized, controlled clinical trials to confirm Avastin's clinical benefit. Avastin's ongoing approval status and Crystal's continued access to Avastin hinged on results from such clinical trials (more on those in a bit).

After Crystal's doctor treated her with Avastin, it took only three months for medical images from MRI, CT, and PET scans to show significant response to therapy. During the Avastin hearing Crystal argued:

> It has been nearly one year now with follow-up scans every three months, and there is currently no evidence of active disease. I'm a testament that the drug does work. Thank God for answered prayers. I've personally had no side effects from Avastin over the last year. Because of my results, I've had more quality time with my family which included seeing my daughter get baptized, taking a vacation to Disney World, attending my brother's wedding, and walking the neighborhood with my parents. Every moment is important to us. Avastin gives us hope. We are counting on the FDA to make the right decision, one that enables all patients, including those newly diagnosed, to have Avastin as an option. Each patient is unique and responds differently. It is morally and ethically wrong to stop treatment for those benefitting. (Avastin hearing transcripts, June 28, 2011, 34–35)[3]

Crystal's testimony was not hyperbole. She contended that, if the breast cancer indication was removed from Avastin's label, her insurance would likely refuse to pay for Avastin—a drug that costs $88,000 a year. Crystal pleaded with her regulatory audience: "If you were me or I was your loved one, wouldn't you want a specialist recommending treatment and the freedom to choose the best options? Please have compassion and value my life. I'm not just a statistic" (Avastin hearing transcripts, June 28, 2011, 35). Crystal's testimony was one of many pro-Avastin arguments made during this hearing and highlights how difficult decision making was because of competing definitions for what counted as clinical benefit.

Once Crystal returned to her seat, Priscilla Howard, another patient diagnosed with metastatic breast cancer, was invited to testify at the microphone. Priscilla described that after being treated with Avastin her doctor told her that she was "progression free, PFS [progression-free survival], but not cancer free" (Avastin hearing transcripts, June 28, 2011, 36). Priscilla went on to remind the FDA that their European counterpart had already determined that Avastin's benefits outweighed the risks. She then asked the FDA, "What endpoint then is sufficient for your approval? Months, years? Despite potential side effects from Avastin, metastatic breast cancer has only one, death. Certainly, Avastin can do no worse" (Avastin hearing transcripts, June 28, 2011, 38).

Pharmaceutical companies (e.g., Genentech) rely on randomized clinical trials (RCTs) to demonstrate clinical benefit. Clinical benefit hinges on a trial's ability to achieve endpoints that are defined by the FDA as "clinically meaningful." So when Priscilla questions the merit of the FDA's preferred endpoint, she is referring to what the FDA defines as "the measurement that will be statistically compared among treatment groups to assess the effect of treatment that corresponds with the clinical trial's objectives, design, and data analysis. For example, a treatment may be tested to decrease the intensity of symptom $Z$. In this case, the endpoint is the change from baseline to time T in a score that represents the concept of symptom $Z$ intensity" (Cappelleri et al. 2013, 8). Priscilla's challenge to the FDA about what endpoints are considered more or less suasive highlights yet again how difficult decision making is in this context due in part to competing criteria for an endpoint's clinical meaningfulness. The FDA's gold standard regarding an endpoint is not progression-free survival. It is overall survival. According to the National Institute of Cancer, overall survival indicates "the percentage of people in a study or treatment group who are still alive for a certain period of time after they were diagnosed with or started treatment for a disease, such as cancer. The overall survival rate is often stated as a five-year survival rate, which is the percentage of people in a study or treatment group who are alive five years after their diagnosis or the start of treatment. Also called survival rate."[4] Because overall survival data are either unavailable or the clinical trial's follow-up time is not long enough according to the FDA, progression-free survival is often used in its place as a surrogate endpoint. Progression-free survival identifies the length of time between a therapeutic intervention and when scans such as PET or MRI suggest that the cancer has advanced (or spread).

Despite moving detail about firsthand experiences with metastatic breast cancer, on June 29, 2011, the FDA voted to remove the breast cancer indication from Avastin's label—a decision that, at the time I write this, has not been overturned.[5] Although Margaret Hamburg (the FDA commissioner at the time of the hearing) acknowledged the evidential value of quality-of-life measures and progression-free survival data in her November 18, 2011, final decision, she argued that these endpoints were simply not meaningful enough to warrant approval for a drug that, while it benefited some, posed grave health risks (e.g., gastrointestinal perforation and fatal bleeding in the stomach and brain) to others who would experience limited or no benefit from Avastin.

The FDA's decision caused uproar from many medical and breast cancer support networks. Discussion among some popular press news outlets summarized the Avastin controversy as "a classic case of data versus anecdote" (Knox 2011, n.p.). Crystal Hanna's testimony that she is "not just a statistic" and Priscilla Howard's challenge to the FDA about an endpoint's suasiveness does seem to suggest the presence of an epistemological chasm between the regulatory world of the FDA and lived experiences of the patients it seeks to protect.

The case of Avastin is the first of its kind. Never before has a drug company challenged the FDA's decision to withdraw approval for a drug after it had been granted accelerated approval. Genentech's challenge was not necessarily driven by big-pharma hubris. Analyses of transcripts from the two-day hearing in June 2011, in addition to previous FDA deliberations and clinical trial data, indicate that there was genuine confusion, disagreement, or at the very least, debate about which endpoint should be considered sufficient as a way to demonstrate clinical benefit. This chapter explores the material-discursive conditions that led to such confusion, disagreement, and debate.[6]

### ASSESSMENT CONUNDRUMS IN THE AVASTIN HEARING

Although changes in laboratory values are considered by the biomedical community to be both objective and superior to the evidence provided by patients (e.g., a patient's answer to questions about how they feel today compared to a month ago), no single endpoint is inherently better or worse than the other. Rather, endpoints articulate implicitly a value judgment about what matters most in a specific cancer-care context. In a *New York Times* article about how medical professionals manage mortality, Dr. Atul Gawande (2014) describes the complexity of what can or ought to be valued in contexts of cancer care. He introduces readers to Peg, a patient who was treated for several years for a rare form of pelvic cancer. Gawande describes the point at which doctors determined very little could be done to improve Peg's cancer diagnosis and prognosis. "This is the moment we continue to debate in our country. What is it we think should happen now? Her condition was incurable by established means. So should she press the doctors for other treatments, experimental therapies, anything with even a remote chance of keeping her going, no matter what? Or should she 'give up'?" (Gawande 2014, n.p.). Gawande is highlighting the complexity inherent in cases like Peg's, a complexity similarly echoed in both Crystal's and Priscilla's testimonies: What endpoints matter most? Overall survival or progression-free survival? Who gets to decide that? And how? During the Avastin hearing one medical professional stalwartly argued that, in fact, "what matters to patients is improvement in overall survival" (Avastin hearing transcripts, June 29, 2011, 175). Patient testimony frequently contradicted such an assertion, however.

Detailed analyses and critique of transcripts from the full Avastin hearing is treated more completely in two previous publications (Teston and Graham 2012; Teston et al. 2014). In this chapter, I mobilize previous findings as exigency for additional analyses of pharmaceutical deliberators' assessment conundrums—in particular, analyses of how cancer researchers' statistical methods both elucidated and limited possibilities for future action. Consensus in the medical community (cf. D'Agostino 2011; Pollack 2010; Twombly 2011) is that the stasis on which the Avastin hearing hinged was not necessarily which endpoint would come to matter most, but which methods were most reliable for measuring an endpoint in the first place. As detailed in the transcripts, deliberations at the Avastin hearing were guided by four overarching questions.

1. Do the ... trials fail to verify the clinical benefit of Avastin for the breast cancer indication for which it was approved?
2. Does the available evidence on Avastin demonstrate that the drug has not been shown to be effective for the breast cancer indication for which it was approved?
3. Does the available evidence on Avastin demonstrate that the drug has not been shown to be safe for the breast cancer indication for which it was approved and that Avastin has not been shown to present a clinical benefit that justifies the risks associated with use of the product for this indication?
4. If the Commissioner agrees with the grounds for withdrawal set out in Issue 1, Issue 2, or Issue 3, should the FDA nevertheless continue the approval of the breast cancer indication while the sponsor designs and conducts additional studies intended to verify the drug's clinical benefit? (Avastin hearing transcripts, June 28, 2011, 10–11)

During their deliberations, expert participants vocalized quite frequently the assessment conundrums posed by cancer researchers' methodological procedures. Such procedures are deliberately designed to help guide answers to each of the above questions.

One FDA deliberator acknowledged "the challenges in powering trials to show statistical significance" and made the case that "the absence of evidence is not evidence of absence. These observations, had they been powered, may—or may not; we can't know for sure—demonstrate a survival advantage" (Avastin hearing transcripts, June 29, 2011, 178). Another FDA deliberator noted, "You can have a statistically significant effect that's not clinically meaningful," but you can also "have a statistically significant effect that is clinically meaningful" (Avastin hearing transcripts, June 29, 2011, 162). Deliberators are grappling with how study design affects whether effects are detected and whether those effects are then deemed significant.

Other FDA deliberators critiqued the clinical trial's method on the basis of measurement: "I think it's very misleading when we always describe treatment effects in a time basis on medians because this is an example, I think, of where the medians are very close, showing .8 months. But actually, there are many points on the curve where the difference is bigger than .8 months. And this actually was seen with a data update that I know that the FDA doesn't rely on" (Avastin hearing transcripts, June 29, 2011, 130). Later in this chapter I explain in greater detail what this deliberator means by describing effects in terms of the passage of time. Important for now, however, is that the methods used to measure an effect and its significance provide the conditions through which patients' disease experiences do or do not warrant possibilities for future action.

The following excerpt provides another example of how statistical methods shape options for future action. "So how can I put a hazard ratio into perspective without looking at the magnitude of the median difference in progression-free survival? ... You can't. You need to look both at hazard ratios and absolute benefits. But I think it's important to look at absolute benefits in time, not just at the median point, but it's the overall separation of the curves. It's early benefits, median benefits, and late benefits" (Avastin hearing transcripts, June 29, 2011, 140–41). These examples are not exhaustive (for that see Teston and Graham 2012; Teston et al. 2014). Rather, they are representative of the overarching assessment conundrums experienced by FDA deliberators during the Avastin hearing. The FDA must reconcile their desire to attune to and make decisions about Avastin's therapeutic efficacy while negotiating the constraints of their primary method for doing so: inferential statistical analyses of survival data. Ultimately, I argue that inferential statistical methods for evidential assessment are one way to attune rhetorically to the presence or absence of disease.[7]

Evidential attunement assumes that we are awash in, entangled among, and partnered with human, nonhuman, and computational coconstructors of the world. Being evidentially attuned, therefore, involves enacting and inhabiting a methodical sensitivity to coconstructors' evidential potentiality, agentic capacity, and ontological suasiveness. Evidential potentiality may be material or immaterial in nature. From stethoscopes to statistical analyses, medical professionals are constantly honing and tinkering with methods for evidential attunement so that they might more readily detect the intricacies of disease and a patient's experience with it. Methodical sensitivity to actors' suasiveness at once shapes and is shaped by what medical professionals finally determine does, in fact, count as evidence of a particular version of or experience with disease. Said simply: evidential potentialities always already exist; methods of evidential attunement animate some potentialities with more argumentative heft than others. The meticulous and methodical nature of evidential attunement in medicine shapes diagnoses, prognoses, and treatment options.

Inferential statistical analysis of survival data sensitizes scientists and medical practitioners to the suasiveness of some evidences, while concomitantly silencing other forms of evidence. In its attempt at isolating real effects from effects that may have nothing at all to do with the intervention under study, inferential statistical analysis can only account for that which can be measured and quantified. For example, although randomization is used as a way to guard against effects stemming from unmeasured and unknown factors, effects from such factors can, in fact, persist. Moreover, inferential statistics flatten both the complexity of laboratories' material methods and patients' bodies, which, as I demonstrated in chapter 2, are in perpetual flux. The method privileges disease experiences that fall within the median response. So while all disease experiences encountered by patients within a clinical trial are a part of the statistical analysis, the very nature of the assessment method forces deliberators to make and justify decisions about efficacy and safety by honing in on median responses.

Deliberators' methodological assessment conundrums invite analysis and critique since some patients who received Avastin saw such an outstanding shrinkage of their tumor and improvement in their cancer and quality of life that researchers and policy makers deemed them super-responders. Both Crystal and Priscilla, for example, were characterized as super-responders. In sum, this means that their bodies' responses to Avastin were not (and could not be) captured by the midpoint of clinical trial results' survival curves. Statistically (and visually), super-responders' experiences lie far outside the survival curve.[8] So while using medians represents more accurately the middle point of a skewed distribution than, say, assessing survival data using means (or averages), its preference for deriving central tendencies minimizes the influence of outlier disease experiences like Crystal's and Priscilla's. And, indeed, this is the very point of inferential statistics: to account for effects at the population level, not at the level of the individual patient. Paradoxically, the suasive power of inferential statistics is also its greatest weakness. I should note that there are different, more innovative ways to analyze survival, but in this particular pharmaceutical hearing, deliberators appear entrenched in inferential statistical analysis as the FDA's standard assessment method (cf. Porter 1996).[9]

In response to the obvious difficulty of having to assess Avastin's efficacy and safety, and given the complexity of the FDA's preferred method for attuning evidentially to cancer (i.e., inferential statistical analyses of survival data), I ask: (1) Are the methodological assessment conundrums present during the FDA's Avastin hearing generalizable to other FDA pharmaceutical hearings (see text box 3.1)? And, (2) if the methodological assessment conundrums at the Avastin hearing are not anomalous, but generalizable to other hearings, how can rhetorical theory help us understand the root cause of such conundrums?

It is my hope that rhetorical theory might help us re-see the complexity of evidential assessment, pharmacological response, and disease experiences in general. A rich, rhetorical understanding of the FDA's current methods for assessing evidence that doesn't seek to place blame or make assumptions about ulterior motives might provide the grounds on which alternative evidences—in particular, those that resist quantification—might, in time, be included in future evidential assessments.[10]

In previous treatments of these data, my coauthors and I asserted that the FDA failed to meaningfully incorporate the testimony of multiple publics (e.g., Crystal Hanna's and Priscilla Howard's), thereby eliding patients' unique, embodied expertise and disease experiences. We acknowledged the possibility that the complexity of the Avastin hearing could have been anomalous but argued that if in subsequent pharmaceutical deliberations the FDA failed to account adequately for nonscientific stakeholders' disease experiences, something had to be done. Otherwise, having an open platform on which members of the public could testify and participate in the hearing is little more than a formal display of feigned inclusion.

My subsequent analyses of FDA pharmaceutical hearings after the 2011 Avastin hearing indicate that both nonexpert and expert deliberators, when faced with the inevitability of a body in flux and cancer's unpredictability, struggle with some of the same assessment conundrums experienced by Avastin hearing deliberators. Results from this study suggest that disagreements concerning the assessment conundrums identified in table 1 are not only characteristic of all pharmaceutical hearings, but such disagreements also occur among and between *expert* participants—not just between expert and nonexpert participants. If assessment conundrums persist even among expert deliberators, and such conundrums are not (only) a function of who gets to speak and whether what they say matters to their audiences, what other suasive actors condition deliberators' decision making?

### ANALYSIS OF POST-AVASTIN PHARMACEUTICAL HEARINGS

*Research Question 1.* Are the methodological assessment conundrums present during the FDA's Avastin hearing generalizable to other FDA pharmaceutical hearings (see table 3.1)?

Since the 2011 Avastin hearing, the FDA has held nineteen pharmaceutical hearings (not involving pediatric pharmaceuticals). Each of these nineteen pharmaceutical hearings lasted somewhere between four and nine hours, and in seventeen of those hearings, a vote was called. Minutes from all hearings are available to the public on the FDA's website. Appendix A provides information about each of the nineteen hearings, which I have distilled into the following identifying features.

- Meeting date and time of hearings.
- Issue, or information about who called the hearing and why. In some cases, a pharmaceutical company did not initiate meetings; rather, the FDA called the meeting to discuss issues related to complexities of an endpoint, methodological approach, or approval status. When the FDA met with the intent of voting on a pharmaceutical intervention, however, they did so because the drug company submitted one of the following: biologics license application, new drug application, supplemental biologics license application, supplemental new drug application.
- The proposed indication that the pharmaceutical company requests the FDA approve. For example, in the case of new drug application #021825 (hearing 3), AcoPharma, Inc., proposed use of Ferriprox to treat patients undergoing chemotherapy whose iron levels are too high. Ten of twelve members voted to approve this indication. As a result, this indication will be added to Ferriprox's drug label.
- The number of nonexpert, public participants who testified at each

hearing. This number ranges from zero nonexpert participants to eighteen participants in hearing 6 wherein Affymax, Inc., proposed that an injection called Peginesatide be used to treat anemia among patients who have been diagnosed with chronic renal failure.

- The primary and secondary endpoints for each of the trials.
- The names of the clinical trials that provide evidence for each hearing.
- The number of members who voted for the proposed indication (indicated by "+"), and the number who voted against (indicated by "–"). Abstentions are also accounted for. Of the seventeen hearings in which votes were called, ten hearings resulted in decisions that favored a pharmaceutical company's proposed indication. Six hearings resulted in a vote that did not favor the proposed indication. The result from hearing 11 is not as easy to determine since seven members voted that the risk/benefit profile was favorable, while four did not, and two abstained.

During five passes through each of the nineteen hearings, I deployed qualitative data analytic moves outlined by Miles and Huberman (1994). These include "affixing" codes, "noting reflections," identifying "similar phrases, relationships," and "patterns, themes, distinct differences between subgroups, and common sequences," and confronting "those generalizations with a formalized body of knowledge in the form of constructs or theories" (9). During the first set of analytic moves, "affixing codes," I relied on Glaser and Strauss's ([1967] 2007) grounded theory approach wherein codes and categories are derived inductively and iteratively. Only after inductively deriving a coding scheme that accounted for the nature of deliberators' debate and disagreement were data introduced to extant rhetorical scholarship as a way of re-seeing how deliberations unfolded during the Avastin hearing.

Based on my analyses of meeting minutes and transcripts, I identified several assessment conundrums in each of the nineteen hearings. For the purposes of this study, I define an assessment conundrum as a moment when debate and disagreement about one or more of the following assessment criteria took place: (1) study design (SD), (2) presence of clinical benefit (CB), (3) reliability and representativeness of data (R), (4) effect size (ES), and (5) risk-benefit ratio (RBR). Table 3.1 provides a list of each of these criteria, the nature of their debate, and examples. The latter half of appendix A provides deliberators' actual stated judgments about the methods used in trials as they were described in each meeting's minutes.

Explicit debate about how researchers designed the clinical trial was

**Table 3.1 Assessment Criteria Debated in Post–Avastin Pharmaceutical Hearings**

| Assessment Criteria | Nature of the Debate | Example |
|---|---|---|
| Study design (SD) | Debate about how the randomized clinical trial (RCT) was designed. | "The single arm design limits the benefit-risk analysis." "Time to event endpoints such as PFS or OS cannot be adequately interpreted in a single-arm trial." "The study was unblinded." |
| Presence of clinical benefit (CB) | Debate about whether a clinically meaningful, positive therapeutic effect could be identified. | "Members who voted no expressed a feeling that the marginal effect demonstrated by the study did not conclusively represent a clinical benefit." "Many members touched on problems with pCR as an endpoint, and uncertainty over whether this translates to long-term clinical benefit for patients." |
| Data reliability or representativeness (R) | Debate about the quality, quantity, reliability, or representativeness of an RCT's data. | "The data is retrospective." "Members who abstained from voting cited a lack of comfort with the quality of the data." "There was limited exposure data in African American populations." |
| Effect size (ES) | Although $p$ values may demonstrate statistical significance, debate ensues about whether the correlation between treatment and its outcome is strong enough. | "Many members stated that the magnitude of improvement in PFS was quite marginal, and was unlikely to be clinically significant, despite having achieved statistical significance." "Members generally agreed that stabilizing these patients to be free of progression was valuable, but that the magnitude of the effect was marginal or modest at best." |
| Risk-benefit ratio (RBR) | Debate about whether risks associated with the treatment outweighs benefits. | "The treatment may be more toxic than the disease itself." "Some members described a discomfort with the definition of deep vein thrombosis in the study." |

coded as study design. Many of the argumentative moves that I coded as SD are remarks regarding the study's single-arm design or unblinded nature. In particular,

- I coded explicit debate about whether a clinically meaningful, positive therapeutic effect could be detected as a concern regarding the presence of clinical benefit. Almost any argumentative move that referenced an effect the deliberator felt was marginal or inconclusive was coded as CB. In general, I coded as CB debate in which "endpoints" were referenced (e.g., "problems with pCR as an endpoint … uncertainty over whether this translates to long-term clinical benefit").
- When deliberators argued about the quality, quantity, reliability, and/or representativeness of the clinical trial's data, I coded such moves as data reliability or representativeness (R). For example, in one hearing, some members abstained from voting on the proposed indication because of their discomfort with the quality or representativeness of the data. In this instance, deliberators were concerned about how the study did not capture data from African American populations. I coded these argumentative moves as R.
- Frequently, deliberations would stall when deliberators tried to assess the relationship between a pharmaceutical treatment and a detected outcome. While $p$ values helped deliberators to determine relationships (since $p$ values indicate strength of relationships), calculating effect size (ES) also helped deliberators resolve this uncertainty (since ES indicates the magnitude of the association or relationship). In vivo utterances that typify this code include "magnitude of effect" and "magnitude of improvement." I coded these argumentative moves as ES.
- Finally, deliberations halted when deliberators argued about whether the risks associated with the pharmaceutical intervention outweighed its benefits. I coded these argumentative moves as risk-benefit ratio (RBR). Representative examples of RBR include: "The treatment may be more toxic than the disease itself" and references to deliberators' "discomfort with the definition of deep vein thrombosis in the study."

Results indicate that the majority of deliberators' post-Avastin debates hinge on how deliberators should regard the very criteria used to assess survival data in the first place.

For example, hearing 19 (app. A) included a proposal for accelerated approval of a drug called Perjeta. The pharmaceutical company (who happens to be Genentech—the same pharmaceutical company that developed the drug discussed earlier in the chapter, Avastin) proposed that Perjeta be added to treatment regimens for patients whose breast cancer diagnosis is considered to be in an early stage but is also aggressive. Genentech argued that Perjeta would help prevent patients' aggressive, early-stage breast cancer from metastasizing (note: the cancer in patients who were treated with Avastin had already metastasized; in a way then, Perjeta posed the potential to prevent the need for Avastin). Although the Perjeta hearing took place more than two years after outcry from the Avastin hearing died down, FDA deliberators had not forgotten about it. In fact, during debate about whether progression-free survival was a suasive endpoint capable of demonstrating clinical benefit, one deliberator in the Perjeta hearing remarked, "We're cautious about that, because we don't, frankly, want another situation like we had with Avastin" (Oncologic Drugs Advisory Committee [ODAC] meeting transcripts, September 12, 2013, 230).[11] Another deliberator argued, "Let's not have a dropdown dog rolling over type of fight, as with Avastin" (ODAC meeting transcripts, September 12, 2013, 275). Disagreement about the clinical meaningfulness of endpoints experienced during the Avastin hearing acted as a kind of rhetorical palimpsest during the Perjeta hearing. Here and in all other deliberations, FDA members grapple with how best to assess the presence, definition, and reliability of evidence. In other words, criteria for assessment were targets of deliberators' interrogations.

One way to theorize the persistence of similar assessment conundrums across all hearings is by characterizing them as "gaps and discoordinations" (Engeström 2001, 76). In an activity theory analysis of general practitioners' work in a health center, gaps and discoordinations are the terms by which Engeström identifies discursively mediated disagreement between patients and doctors.[12] For Engeström, these gaps and discoordinations elucidate "certain aspects of the 'invisible work' going on in all work settings" (76). Persistent assessment conundrums (or gaps and discoordinations) point to the presence of some type of unaccounted for, invisible, backstage labor. Graham and Herndl (2013) noted similar gaps and discoordinations in their analyses of differences between pain management practitioners and other medical practitioners and initially wondered about the applicability of Feyerabend's incommensurability when characterizing such differences. In place of (what they see as) the limiting rhetorical and practical consequences of Feyerabendian incommensurability, Graham and Herndl (2013) offer an alternative theory: Annemarie Mol's (2002) multiple ontologies, which they define as a "postplural model for inquiry into rhetoric of science" (103). Mol's theory of multiple ontologies helps us steer clear of (the sometimes unproductive) interrogations about the nature of interlocutors' disagreement; in so doing, we can then pursue questions about the problem's origin (Graham and Herndl 2013, 123).

The remainder of my analysis, therefore, takes up an account of how evidential conundrums persist—but not by asking, "about what do FDA experts and nonexpert members of the public disagree?" Rather, borrowing from Graham and Herndl, I ask, "From where does the problem come?" Exploring the persistence of FDA assessment conundrums in this way permits an investigative detour around the trap that Condit (2013) calls "science bad" or "science too powerful" (2) studies.

### UNDERSTANDING PROBABILITY AS *POESIS*

*Research Question 2.* What does rhetorical theory offer us as we attempt to understand the root cause of the FDA's assessment conundrums?

One key finding from the above analyses is that assessment conundrums encountered by deliberators in the Avastin hearing were not anomalous. Both experts and nonexperts alike in all subsequent pharmaceutical hearings struggled with how conditions of assessment criteria themselves ought to be regarded. In the remainder of this chapter, then, I locate at the seat of method the place from where assessment conundrums of pharmaceutical deliberations hail. I argue that the persistence of evidential assessment conundrums is rooted in the real and material effects of cancer researchers' methods for assessing probability. Probabilistic methods for assessing data both create and constrain assessment possibilities. Probabilistic assessments do rhetorical work, therefore. Although hidden from plain sight in the biomedical backstage, such methods have a hand in how cancer treatments are approved or not.

Making inferences about the efficacy and safety of cancer treatments requires members of the FDA to engage in probabilistic assessments. Deliberators must take what is known presently and render from those available data an argument about what is not yet known. Inferential statistics is contemporary cancer researchers' primary strategy for bringing forth or bringing out of concealment into unconcealment, in a Heideggerian (1977) sense, the likelihood that an intervention will be effective not just for patients enrolled in a clinical trial but for other patients as well.[13] Although the Greeks did not have a numbering system that allowed them to engage in probabilistic reasoning, their term for making—*poesis*—aptly captures the nature of probability as a method of material making that has real consequences for cancer care.

## Probability's Suasiveness

Miller (2003) posits that decisions like those made by the FDA—decisions that rely on "formal method ... numbers and algorithms" are believed to be "both fairer and truer than those based on experiential judgment because their impersonality is interpreted as objectivity" (196). For Miller, "Quantification can be seen as a form of expertise that is independent of experts" (196). This may be why in FDA pharmaceutical hearings we see assessment-related gaps and discoordinations across a range of expertise: The only true expert in the room is the probabilistic method itself.[14]

Miller (2003) makes the very astute observation that quantification "assists ethos in its concealment as logos" (196). Similarly, in an earlier argument, Porter (1996) notes that "a decision made by the numbers (or by explicit rules of some other sort) has at least the appearance of being fair and impersonal. Scientific objectivity thus provides an answer to a moral demand for impartiality and fairness. Quantification is a way of making decisions without seeming to decide. Objectivity lends authority to officials who have very little of their own" (8). Both Miller (2003) and Porter (1996) characterize the argumentative power of decisions made by numbers as rooted in its impersonality.

When I attempt to extend this argument into probabilistic assessments performed by the FDA, however, I see that deliberators do not assume that their probabilistic assessments are unburdened by the weight of outside influences and external contributors. That is, it's quite clear from the above analyses that FDA deliberators are keenly aware of how probabilistic methods are neither impersonal nor objective. Statistical methods used in FDA pharmaceutical hearings help assess survival data, but evidential certainty is hampered by the fact that such methods are *not* impartial contributors to medical decision making. Rather, deliberators understand that probabilistic methods for assessing survival data possess the power to shape options for future action well enough on their own.[15]

The idea that methods of probabilistic assessment frame conditions and criteria for decision making is not a new insight. Kahneman and Tversky (1984) illustrated probability's suasive power in their description of physicians' and patients' assessment of risk when given the otherwise equally effective treatment options of either radiation or surgery. Kahneman and Tversky found that a patient's decision hinged on how the physician framed the choice in terms of mortality or survival. Patients seemed to know implicitly that surgery always entails risk of death while radiation therapy, in contrast, does not. Consequently, "the surgery option was relatively less attractive when the statistics of treatment outcomes were described in terms of mortality rather than in terms of survival" (Kahneman and Tversky 1984, 346). The authors conclude that when options for future action are framed in terms of loss or death, probability of risk "looms larger than gains" (346). Kahneman and Tversky's illustration takes us only so far in our desire to understand from where assessment gaps and discoordinations hail, however. Indeed, discursive framing of probabilities is meaningful and helps to bring forth (or bring out of concealment into unconcealment) possibilities for future action. But in Kahneman and Tversky's illustration, "the overall difference in life expectancy was not great enough to provide a clear choice between the two forms of treatment" (Bernstein 2003, 276). In the case of the Avastin hearing (and all subsequent pharmaceutical hearings), choices were, indeed, different, and their discursive frames barely account for the complexity of those differences. How, then, do we account for probability's argumentative affordances that, aside from discursive frames, make salient some choices (and frames), but not others?

Clinically meaningful endpoints such as progression-free survival or overall survival may be discursive frames for describing effects, but endpoints are more than markers for bad versus good options. On their own, endpoints are mere numbers that enable probability-based arguments; but once they're mobilized within a decision-making context, they confer a host of material biases—biases that are glossed over discursively by words like, "meaningful," "progression-free," and even "survival." There are real, material, backstage conditions that render such discursive frames possible.

## Probability's Materiality

One way to understand how backstage material methods condition probability's suasiveness is to examine methods' making-power. To prepare readers for forthcoming analyses of probability's material making-power, consider that premodern probability was rendered, quite literally, through material objects. Paleolithic probability practices, in particular, involved tossing a running animal's knucklebone, or talus. "In creatures such as deer, horse, oxen, sheep and hartebeest this bone is so formed that when it is thrown to land on a level surface it can come to rest in only four ways. Well polished and often engraved examples are regularly found on the sites of ancient Egypt.... Similar sheep-like tali begin to occur on Sumerian and Assyrian sites. Well polished, oft-used knucklebones are found even in the Paleolithic dwellings" (Hacking 1975, 1–2). In fact, some scholars argue that premodern probability relied on tali without "a set of four equal chances. Moreover, the distribution of chances varies from talus to talus according to the distribution of mass in the heelbone" (Hacking 1975, 4). Hacking, however, maintains that after spending an afternoon rolling dice located in the cabinets of the Cairo Museum of Antiquities, he found that there were "plenty of stochastically sound Fundamental Probability Sets to be had in ancient times" (4). Nevertheless, Hacking's heel bone–turned-die hypothesis invites considerations of how probabilities are material constructions whose stochastic soundness is never guaranteed. Rickert (2013), drawing on Heidegger (1977), similarly argues, "every unconcealing is also a concealing" (175).

To understand the role of statistical methods for constructing probability, one must consider more than discursive or visual renderings. In a Toulminian sense, discursive articulations of statistical probabilities akin to Kahneman and Tversky's (1984) frames are mere qualifiers—they help to assert implicitly or explicitly the strength of a claim about an intervention's effectiveness. In the clinical decision-making moment, patients are constrained by having access only to the limited nature of discursive qualifiers. And how could they be provided with anything more substantial? Argumentative grounds and backing (again, in a Toulminian sense) on which a statistical probability is rendered includes black-boxed, discipline-specific calculations.

The task for technical communicators and rhetoricians, therefore, is to at once unhinge and also account for evidential assessments' entanglements between humans, visual and discursive representations, statistical methods of analyses, and probabilistic renderings. Only in doing so do we have any hope of moving beyond the discursive battlefield described at this chapter's outset—a battlefield wherein those who wield the dominance of a discourse always already gain the adherence of minds (Perelman and Olbrechts-Tyteca 1969). Again, "rhetoric is not exclusively a symbolic art, nor does it issue solely from human being. Rhetoric is fundamentally wedded to the world and emerges within that world. Rhetoric is a modality of the world's revealing itself, including human being" (Rickert 2013, 176). If we have any hope of understanding from where a problem comes during periods of medical uncertainty, particularly when competing assessments of risk collide (as in the case of the Avastin hearing), we must begin by understanding method as a rich space for making, doing, and being—a space where human being and the world are intricately woven.

To model such a task, and explore in greater detail probability's material conditions with and through which deliberators make and do, in this next section, I explore from where disagreements originate by demonstrating how the very thing responsible for what *can* be known at FDA pharmaceutical hearings is also responsible for that which *cannot*. While inferential statistics presents several argumentative affordances insofar as it is able to distinguish noise from evidential signal, it simultaneously imposes rigid assessment boundaries between that which can and cannot (not necessarily should or should not) be detected as data in the first place.

## UNDERSTANDING INFERENTIAL
## STATISTICS AS ENTHYMEMATIC

I suggested in chapter 1 that rhetoric is doing, or a way of performing the world materially (Barad 2007, 335). What, then, can we learn about inferential statistics when we frame it as rhetoric? Since "phenomena are not the result merely of human laboratory contrivances or human concepts" but "are specific material performances of the world" (Barad 2007, 335), it stands to reason that cancer researchers and scientists are not lone agentic actors, and mathematics is not a mere tool they wield to make an argument. So, then, how exactly *does* inferential statistics make possible an assessment of bodies' locatable-for-now coordinates? How do probabilistic methods in general and inferential statistics in particular attune deliberators to some ways of seeing certain kinds and forms of evidence, but not others? How does inferential statistics as a method of evidential attunement "bring the world into rhetorical performance" (Rickert 2013, xviii)? How does inferential statistics animate some material realities and not others? To explore these questions, I zoom in on the enthymematic nature of Kaplan-Meier tactics for statistical analysis and mobilize rhetorical theory's enthymeme as a construct capable of accounting for the suasive properties of inferential statistics.

I am not the first to note the ontological relationship between statistics and enthymemes. Making statistical inferences, as Macdonald (2004) has argued, "involves reasoning on the basis of incomplete information and does not lead to necessary conclusions" (193). Here, Macdonald makes the case that, just as Aristotelian enthymemes are incomplete syllogisms, so too are statistical tests, which "involves inferring from a set of data that the direction of an observed difference cannot plausibly by attributed to chance" (195). Moreover, "reasoning from probability models involves reasoning on the basis of an analogy" (Macdonald 2004, 202). As an assessment method, inferential statistics employs a host of tactics for distilling data from noise and defining boundaries between what will or will not be included in the analysis itself. Such a method renders quantitative order from biological chaos.

To assess clinical trial data, deliberators and inferential statisticians ask: How likely is it that we would have observed what we observed (or something even more extreme) from this same, exact study population outside of the boundaries of the study, itself? From there, inferential statisticians must also ask whether the findings from this patient sample are likely to be true about other patients. And then, patients, along with their support team, must determine for themselves whether the findings from this sample population are likely to be true for them. Biases and chance influence how answers to these questions are resolved. I characterize inferential statistical analysis as an enthymematic enterprise because of the chain of statistical premises that condition and structure the answers to those questions. In an effort to account for bias and chance, cancer researchers and FDA deliberators calculate and posit a chain of statistical premises in the form of hazard ratios, confidence intervals, effect size, and $p$ values.

Inferential statistics yields best guesses about a patient population that, because it is logistically impossible to include an entire population of interest in a given trial, cannot (and never will) be available for analysis. Best guesses and estimates are based on what occurs when smaller samples of such a population are studied. For example, when FDA deliberators in the Avastin hearing use inferential statistics to analyze a patient's survival probability, they're estimating probabilities for a futuristic, imaginary patient population that has not yet taken a particular drug or been diagnosed with a particular cancer. To make best guesses about a population that is not yet ready to hand, inferential statistical analysis generalizes findings from a representative sample to that of a larger, as of yet unavailable population. According to Burnyeat (1996), Aristotle's enthymeme is a "deduction that can be applied to contexts where conclusive proof is not to be had" (99). In Scott's (2002) enthymematic analysis of public policy debates surrounding newborn HIV testing, he opens by comparing the typical definition of enthymeme—"truncated syllogism[s] based on probable rather than certain premises" (57)—to Jeffrey Walker's definition: "Drawing mainly from Isocrates, Walker describes the enthymeme as a body of persuasion that presents a claim, foregrounds a stance, and motivates identification with this stance by invoking a chain of premises and a cluster of value-charged proofs" (57). Scott then invokes John Gage's (1991) definition of an enthymeme as an "'architectonic rhetorical structure valuable in the invention process,' a heuristic for 'discovering the *best* reasons'" (2002, 57). Enthymemes are, therefore, more than truncated syllogisms. Reliant on a chain of premises, enthymemes have heuristic power. And more than that, according to Scott: "An enthymeme entails not only a generative structure for an argument but also the argument itself" (58). Having limited access only to clinical trial data from a smaller sample of a much larger potential population, deliberators must make inferences using enthymematic reasoning about how a treatment will affect the survival rates of a larger population. Deliberators make such inferences using a chain of premises made up of statistical probabilities rendered from analyses of smaller, immediately available populations.

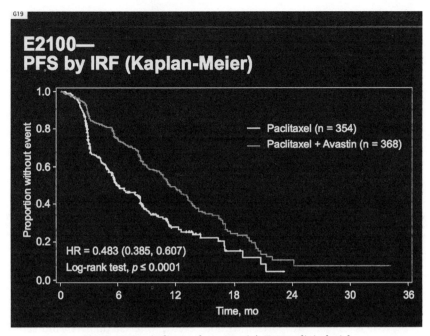

Figure 3.1 Survival curve from Avastin's E2100 clinical trial

Inferential statistical analysis is enthymematic on both a macro and micro level. At the macro level, claims about a drug's efficacy are rooted in the rhetorical strategy of making a larger claim based on the strength and magnitude of that same claim in a smaller population. At the micro level, such population-level claims can only be made when warranted by specific chains of premises and proofs. As an illustration of how inferential statistical analysis is enthymematic on both the macro and micro level, consider the case of one of Avastin's clinical trials, E2100. In E2100, 685 patients were monitored after being placed (through randomization) in one of two treatment arms. From this sample population, Genentech made broader, more generalizable claims about the drug's safety and efficacy. This is the first instance of enthymematic argumentation. Genentech researchers and analysts partnered with inferential statistical methods to analyze data from a clinical trial, the results of which were generalized to a larger population. Deliberators visually displayed during the Avastin hearing such results in the form of a survival curve (see fig. 3.1).

To graphically show survival curves, statisticians used what is called Kaplan-Meier analysis. In 1958, collaborators Edward Kaplan and Paul Meier developed this method as a way to make claims about a study population when observations may not be complete for one reason or another (see Rich et al. [2010] for more background on this method). The Kaplan-Meier method allows researchers to make survival estimates by filling in the gaps left by patients who may have had to drop out of the study. Claims are made within the Kaplan-Meier statistical method in the form of survival rates and hazard rates. A survival rate is, as one might guess, the probability that a patient will survive beyond an agreed on time (i.e., $p[T > t]$). The hazard ratio, in contrast, is *not* a time-based measure. Rather, hazard ratios assess the chance that an event (e.g., death, remission) will occur in a study's treatment arm divided by the chance that same event will occur in the control arm (or vice versa).

As illustrated in figure 3.1, patients involved in the trial were monitored over the span of three years, or thirty-six months. In total, 368 patients received Avastin in this study. Patients who received Avastin in addition to a drug called Paclitaxel make up one treatment arm, while the other treatment arm included patients who were treated only with Paclitaxel. The survival curve in figure 3.1 is a final visual representation of survival data; progression-free survival is the primary endpoint in this particular analysis. The $y$ axis is labeled "Proportion without event," wherein an event indicates the spread, or advancement, of cancer as can be detected pathologically or radiologically. (For more on how medical professionals partner with medical visualizations to manage biomedical indeterminacy, see chap. 2.) As the survival curve illustrates, patients who received Avastin clearly lived longer without advancement (or an event) in their disease.

During the E2100 trial, an independent radiology facility (or "IRF," as indicated in figure 3.1) analyzed these data using inferential statistics, and results from their analysis can be found in figure 3.2—another slide displayed during the Avastin hearing. As demonstrated in the far right column of figure 3.2, of the 368 patients who were treated with Avastin, 173 of them experienced some advancement in their disease (or death) during the trial. This amounts to 47 percent of that sample population. Of the 354 patients who *did not* receive Avastin during the clinical, 184 patients, or 52 percent of that sample, experienced the spread of their disease. By these measures, it would seem that the addition of Avastin resulted in a slight treatment advantage over Paclitaxel alone.

Even if in the best of circumstances patients are provided with survival probabilities and concomitant inferences about whether certain treatments might benefit them, how such probabilities and inferences came to be are black-boxed (Latour 1987). Rhetorical theory can help unearth how survival probabilities are rendered methodologically in the biomedical backstage.

# E2100—
# PFS by Independent Radiology Facility (IRF)

| | Paclitaxel (n = 354) | Paclitaxel + Avastin (n = 368) |
|---|---|---|
| Patients with an event, n (%) | 184 (52) | 173 (47) |
| Stratified analysis | | |
| HR | 0.483 | |
| 95% CI | (0.385, 0.607) | |
| p value | | |
| Log-rank | < 0.0001 | |
| PFS, mo | | |
| Median | 5.8 | 11.3 |
| 95% CI | (5.36, 8.15) | (10.45, 13.27) |

Figure 3.2 Results from statistical analysis in Avastin's E2100 clinical trial

Clearly, visual representations of survival data vis-à-vis Kaplan-Meier survival curves tell only one part of the assessment story. So, what about the very probabilities on which survival curves are constructed? What enthymematic premises condition how inferential statistical methods do argumentative work?

Argumentative contributors to inferential statistics include a chain of enthymematic premises—specifically, hazard ratios, confidence intervals, effect size, and $p$ values. Each inferential premise attunes deliberators to see or assess data differently. As a method, inferential statistics mobilizes enthymematic premises in ways that have real, material effects on medical professionals' assessments. That is, the enthymematic premises of inferential statistics make more or less suasive certain disease experiences. At the same time that inferential statistics detects and accounts for the material conditions of a patient population's disease experiences, the method's materiality itself shapes what can and cannot (yet) be detected.

Before I describe with more specificity how inferential statistics' enthymematic premises shape what can and cannot be detected, I must clarify that inferential statistics as a method is designed to either reject or fail to reject what is called the null hypothesis. The null hypothesis is a researcher's default position that in the case of Avastin, for example, asserts that there is no difference between the patients who *did* receive Avastin and the patients who *did not* receive Avastin. If a researcher rejects the null hypothesis, he or she has grounds to make the argument that, within the parameters of a particular study (i.e., Avastin's E2100 clinical trial), Avastin may, in fact, have had a statistically significant effect. If a researcher fails to reject the null hypothesis (which indicates that a measurable difference between the treatment and control arms could not be detected), he or she can thereby infer that Avastin did not have a statistically significant effect.

The potential for error in clinical trials always exists, however. Inferential statistics' enthymematic premises help (but never fully) clarify the likelihood that researchers have committed what statisticians refer to as type I or type II errors. A type I error, which is represented by the Greek letter alpha ($\alpha$), indicates a false positive. A type I error occurs when researchers falsely reject the default position that Avastin, for example, did not have a treatment effect. Said another way: type I errors occur when the biomedical backstage has in some way managed to produce spurious, significant differences between treatment and control arms. Type II errors ($\beta$), conversely, are false negatives. Type II errors occur when researchers mistakenly fail to reject the default position that Avastin, for example, has had no treatment effect. In other words, when a type II error occurs, the biomedical backstage has in some way managed to obscure what should have been an otherwise statistically significant difference between treatment and control arms. Notable here is that, in inferential statistics, researchers want to be able to *reject* the null hypothesis. In so doing, they are rejecting the premise that there was not a treatment effect. Researchers can, therefore, make the logical leap that there was, in fact, a treatment effect. However, to make that logical leap requires several assumptions about the biomedical backstage.

First, when declaring that a treatment had no effect, one must assume that scientists were capable of detecting the effect in the first place. Second, one must assume that detection and measurement are synonymous. So, for example, in an earlier draft of this chapter, the previous paragraphs at one time included the phrase "no measurable effect" until a colleague and biomedical statistician advised that I delete the word "measurable." The assumption implicit in deleting "measurable" is that (*a*) effects that might be meaningful are detectable in the biomedical backstage, and (*b*) we have the material means and methods by which to measure such effects. In the case of Avastin, inferential statistics is not designed to permit a hypothesis that states, "Avastin will have an effect." Although the logical leap is made to claim that there was, in fact, a treatment effect when the null hypothesis is rejected, its rejection does not permit a researcher to claim with certainty that a particular drug is, in fact, responsible for an effect. Any and all claims about an effect must be made probabilistically; and such probabilities hinge on a chain of enthymematic premises—premises I will now describe in greater detail.

### Hazard-Based versus Time-Based Measures

When looking to make arguments about a patient's survival probability, medical professionals and scientists assess clinical trial data using hazard-based and/or time-based measures. Differences between the two types of measures have an effect on how researchers assess the results of their clinical trial. Relying on hazard-based measures requires a researcher to estimate differences in hazard rates between treatment and control arms. Hazard rates are probabilistic assessments that support (or not) an assertion that, if an event (e.g., death) has not already occurred, it will, in fact, occur in the next instance of time. A hazard rate expresses the probability that, for example, if a patient has not died in ten years, he or she will die in the next instance of time (e.g., a second later). Again, hazard rates are probabilistic, not fixed and finite predictions.

Time-based measures, in contrast, require the researcher to rely on either group medians or means to assess when a patient might experience a particular event (e.g., death, remission)—again, such an assessment is probabilistic. If a researcher chooses to rely on time-based measures and decides that medians will be the best indicator of a patient's survival probability, he or she is making the decision to value as evidence the time about which 50 percent of cases are said to experience a particular event (e.g., death, remission). Researchers decide ahead of time what "experiencing a particular event" means. If, for example, a researcher decides ahead of time that death is the event on which a time-based measure will hinge, and that medians are more reliable than means in this case, the researcher calculates when, during the course of the clinical trial, approximately 50 percent of participants pass away.

Alternatively, the researcher might opt instead to rely on group means instead of medians as their assessment parameter. Unlike group medians (which highlight the time at which 50 percent of cases are resolved), group means calculate study participants' average time to event (e.g., death, remission) and is represented by the area under the Kaplan-Meier curve. The choice to use either medians or means as the primary time-based measure can drastically shape how data are assessed—especially in the case of Avastin when some patients (i.e., Crystal and Priscilla described at the beginning of this chapter) were characterized as super-responders. Super-responders' hazard-based and time-based measures were so drastically different from the norm that they could skew the distribution. This is precisely why medians (not means) are used to describe survival. When describing population survivals, it is undesirable to allow outlier data to influence such descriptions.

Spruance et al. (2004) illustrate the difference between hazard-based versus time-based measurements in terms of a race—specifically, "the difference between hazard-based and time-based measures is analogous to the odds of winning a race and the margin of victory" (2791). In Spruance et al.'s illustration, hazard-based measures are analogous to whether a participant has crossed the finish line, while time-based measures are analogous to the winner's margin of victory. In the case of Avastin, one might map these different measures onto the following two questions: If the patient is treated with Avastin, how likely is it (when compared with patients from the control arm) that their cancer will not have spread? versus, if the patient is treated with Avastin, by what day, week, or month is it likely that their cancer will have spread? Hazard ratios versus time-based measures facilitate two different ways of seeing and thereby assessing the same pool of data. So as not to be swayed by the making-power of one over the other, during deliberations, hazard ratios and time-based measures are evaluated together.

### Confidence Intervals

Another premise on which enthymematic arguments in inferential statistical analyses are made is the confidence interval. Confidence intervals are expressed as a range between two numbers. The formal definition of a confidence interval is: "a range of values that measure a treatment effect that are constructed so that this range has a specified probability of including the true value of the variable" (Davies and Crombie 2009, 4). In other words, confidence intervals point to the probability that a "true" treatment effect will fall within a specific range. For example, in figure 3.2, Avastin researchers calculated that 95 percent of the time, the hazard ratio (discussed in the previous section) will fall somewhere between 0.385 and 0.607 (as a reminder: hazard ratios are a calculation of the relationship between the treatment arm's hazard rate versus the control group's hazard rate). Conventionally, researchers assume that 95 percent of the time "properly constructed confidence intervals should contain the true value of the variable of interest.... More colloquially, the confidence interval provides a range for our best guess of the size of the true treatment effect that is plausible given the size of the difference actually observed" (Davies and Crombie 2009, 4). Confidence intervals, therefore, enact an a priori agreement about where researchers' analytic boundaries lie.

Confidence intervals are not impervious to a study's material conditions, however. For example, the size of the sample that researchers study affects confidence intervals, as does the degree of difference between variables within that sample. So, if a population is quite small, the research is more likely to detect an effect—an effect that may or may not be "true." Small population sizes, therefore, can affect or bias confidence intervals. Conversely, a clinical trial whose population is quite large may make it difficult for researchers to detect effects; perhaps if the population were slightly smaller, such always already existing effects could not be so easily glossed over or go undetected. Studies that have larger populations tend to result in narrower confidence intervals—that is, the degree of difference between the two numbers is smaller. Generally speaking, it is desirable to have narrower confidence intervals, as a wider range between confidence intervals may suggest the study was imprecise. In other words, if the gap between the two confidence limits is large, researchers may interpret this to mean that the study was designed (or what one deliberator in the Avastin hearing referred to as "powered") in such a way to capture a wide range of effects—some of which may not be true.

Statisticians are well aware of how study design shapes results and as such have tried to mitigate type I or type II errors by attuning to another calculation: statistical power. In essence, statistical power refers to the likelihood that, for example, researchers in Avastin's E2100 clinical trial successfully designed the study in such a way to detect an effect if there is an effect to be detected. The makers of Avastin, Genentech, understand that pharmaceutical clinical trials are expensive. Mindful of this, cancer researchers make decisions about how to design their study in a way that errs on the side of committing a type II error. In the case of a low-stakes pharmaceutical intervention, researchers may design the study (or bias it) so that if there is an error to be made, at least the error will be one that fails to reject the null hypothesis. Alternatively, when researchers work with a high-stakes pharmaceutical intervention (e.g., Avastin), they may design the study so that it is biased toward obtaining false positives, since such findings would yield greater financial opportunity.

### Effect Size

Thus far, I've only described inferential statistics' making-power in terms of whether a researcher can detect an effect. But statisticians also account for *ranges* of effects. Range of effect is yet another enthymematic premise that indicates the study design's attunement to some disease experiences, or evidences, over others. Effect sizes help researchers ensure that the thing they're actually measuring is the thing they want (or intended) to measure.

In the case of Avastin, for example, the effect size allows researchers to assert whether the way they've designed their study has made it possible for them to attune to Avastin's ineffectuality among certain populations. Moreover, effect size helps assure the researcher that he or she isn't measuring an external artifact that may skew or obfuscate attunement to Avastin's ineffectuality among certain populations. Respectable and reliable decision making hinges heavily on effect size as an enthymematic premise since, without it, it is possible to detect an effect that is statistically significant, but one never knows if that effect is due to something other than the intervention under investigation.

Concerns about effect size indicate how difficult it is to isolate intervention-related effects from outside, ambient contributors. For example, in Genentech's Avastin E2100 clinical trial, without knowing the study's effect size, it is difficult to determine if Avastin is the reason participants in the treatment arm look different than participants in the control group. If participants in one treatment arm have an event (e.g., death, stroke) for reasons unrelated either to having received Avastin or to having cancer (e.g., car accident, skydiving accident), researchers make every effort to censor these data so as not to skew the effect size.

Effect sizes are useful in that they make possible comparisons to other things within the study or across similar studies (e.g., meta-analyses). Typically, researchers determine ahead of time what an acceptable or unacceptable effect size is, but that parameter matters most when it is placed in relationship to the other enthymematic premises described above.

### p Values

Unlike some of the other enthymematic premises introduced above, readers may be more familiar with or at least aware of the suasive power of a p value. These values are calculated as a way to assess the probability that results of a clinical trial are due to chance and not to the effect an intervention had on participants in the study's treatment arm. These probabilistic calculations are made with the assumption that the clinical trial was well conducted. The p value indicates whether, for instance, Genentech's researchers can claim that their findings in Avastin's E2100 study are statistically significant.

The conventional cutoff point for determining whether findings are statistically significant is equal to or less than .05. That is, if the p value is calculated as less than .05, the trial's results are considered statistically significant. If a p value is calculated as greater than .05, questions about the statistical significance of the trial's findings ensue. In a two-tailed test—that is, a test wherein researchers are looking for differences in either direction—the $p$ value limit is .025, but statisticians still employ an alpha of .05. In the future, researchers at Genentech might make a case that the alpha value ought to be .10 or .25. By changing the alpha value, researchers permit attunement to more possible effects; in so doing, however, researchers' confidence that those effects are truly different from what might occur simply by chance is lessened.

In inferential statistics, $p$ values help researchers know if a treatment group's outperformance of a control group is real or a chance finding. And yet, a $p$ value greater than .05 (which indicates the lack of statistical significance) does not necessarily mean that the intervention under study failed to produce an effect. In fact, when a clinical trial has fewer participants, it's quite likely that researchers will be unable to achieve statistical significance even if or when there may very well be real and important effects. In other words, if that study had been designed to include more participants, researchers may have been able to more readily detect an effect that resulted in a lower $p$ value, thereby indicating statistical significance. Conversely, a $p$ value less than .05 (which indicates that there *is* statistical significance) does not necessarily mean the effect is real.

Finally, and perhaps most importantly, statistical significance—a simple number that seems to say a lot—does not always correspond directly with that which is clinically meaningful. The tension between the argumentative heft of a study's $p$ value versus the study's effect size was especially pertinent in the case of Avastin. Clinical meaningfulness is best captured by effect size, not necessarily the presence of statistical significance.

Recall that the null hypothesis of inferential statistics asserts that there is no (measurable) difference between treatment and control arms. Calculating $p$ values requires only the option to reject the null hypothesis. In other words, the question that the $p$ value answers is: How likely is it that we have observed a difference between the control and treatment arm simply because of chance and not because of our pharmaceutical intervention's effect? Davies and Crombie (2009) put it this way:

> The $p$-value is the probability that we would observe effects as big as those seen in the study if there was really no difference between the treatments. If $p$ is small, the findings are unlikely to have arisen by chance and we reject the idea that there is no difference between the two treatments (we reject the null hypothesis). If $p$ is large, the observed difference is plausibly a chance finding and we do not reject the

idea that there is no difference between the treatments. Note that we do not reject the idea, but we do not accept it either: we are simply unable to say one way or another until other facts have been considered. (2)

Again, *p* values are considered small if they are less than .05. If a *p* value is less than .05, this means that there is a "less than one in 20 chance that a difference as big as that seen in the study could have arisen by chance if there was really no true difference" (Davies and Crombie 2009, 2). In the case of Genentech's Avastin E2100 clinical trial, the *p* value is considered highly significant. This means that when patients received Avastin alongside another drug, Paclitaxel, the effects were highly statistically significant with regard to patients' progression-free survival. But the range of effects, or effect size—not the *p* value—tipped the argumentative balance for some deliberators, as did the fact that these effect sizes are less suasive when you change the primary endpoint from progression-free survival to overall survival.

In sum, the Kaplan-Meier survival curve in figure 3.1 tells only a fraction of the analytic story. What I have tried to do here is unfold the flatness or two-dimensionality of the survival curves displayed during the Avastin hearing in the hope that even nonstatisticians can see how hazard ratios, confidence intervals, effect sizes, and *p* values help to coconstruct deliberators' final evidential assessments. Such contributors act as enthymematic premises by exerting making-power in the biomedical backstage. Inferential statistical analyses of clinical trial data hinge on the making-power of each enthymematic premise. Inferential statistical analysis is a rhetorical act inasmuch as it involves a series of intra-actions between enthymematic premises—premises on which final claims are assessed as more or less accurate, significant, and meaningful.

This chapter opens the black box of how inferential statistical analysis attunes deliberators to value some degrees of disease experiences or evidence over others. Evidential assessments like those made by the FDA in the Avastin hearing hinge not only on technical and expert parameters of how, for example, endpoints are deemed more or less meaningful, but also on the statistical partnerships that attune deliberators to bioinformation's meaningfulness in the first place.

I present these findings not to suggest that they alone have the power to change the outcome of public policies akin to those made by the FDA in Genentech's Avastin hearing. I am not even suggesting that the outcome of the Avastin hearing should have been different. In fact, it may be that things are as they should be. The contentious nature of the FDA's deliberations and their method for incorporating public participation in policy making garnered a good deal of attention from news media and various stakeholder groups. Increased attention to the machinations of evidential assessments in public policy scenarios is, to my mind, desirable. Rather, my analyses of evidential attunements deployed in the biomedical backstage long before the actual Avastin hearing itself offer a rich and relevant example of how deliberative decision making and public policy is frequently performed materially backstage, well prior to formal, discursive, or deliberative moments. When evidences collide or compete (e.g., so-called data versus anecdote [Knox 2011, n.p.]) decisions hinge on the biomedical backstage's evidential attunements.

Arguing that "rhetoric is not, finally, a shift in the mental states of subjects but something world-transforming for individuals and groups immersed in vibrant, ecologically attuned environments" (xv), Rickert (2013) draws analytic attention to ambient contributors to human being. He argues that the "theoretical move from rhetorical subjects to ambient environments" necessitates a "move to ontological rather than epistemic considerations," thereby "shifting conversations away from . . . issues of truth and falsehood or the problem of knowledge versus opinion" (xvi), or in the case of pharmaceutical hearings, "data versus anecdote" (Knox 2011, n.p.). Understanding how methods for assessing evidences attune deliberators in particular ways is useful to any party who participates in cross-disciplinary, cross-expertise negotiations of meaning, being, and, in the case of managing biomedical indeterminacy, surviving.

### ATTUNING TO AND ASSESSING OTHER EVIDENCES

Observing that public participation at the Avastin hearing made little to no difference in the final outcome of the hearing originally led my coauthors and I to surmise that the FDA's elided breast cancer survivors' testimony because they lacked expertise (Teston and Graham 2012; Teston et al. 2014). We distilled the argumentative disconnect (or gaps, discoordinations, and incommensurability) into a reductive assertion about the difference between anecdotal and statistical evidences. However, my analyses of pharmaceutical hearings held post-Avastin indicate that assessment conundrums are not unique to the complexity of Genentech's Avastin hearing. In all subsequent pharmaceutical hearings (excluding pediatric pharmaceutical hearings, which were not analyzed), similar evidential assessment conundrums abound. Moreover, even expert deliberators grappled with questions about the best way to assess clinical trial data.

To counter the absurd possibility that Schrödinger's cat would be smeared out in equal parts, Barad (2007) argues that on opening the box, we will find the cat either dead or alive, not in some in-between state. She concludes that "*measurement resolves the indeterminacy*" (280; italics in the original). Specifically, "when we observe a system, it ceases to be in a superposition. But how is the indeterminacy resolved? By what mechanism does the system go from a superposition of eigenstates to a definite value measured for the corresponding property?" (280). For Barad, unknowability or indeterminacy is resolved as a result of material mechanisms for measurement, of which inferential statistical analysis is but one.

Inferential statistics does work or performs rhetorically because its chain of enthymematic premises lends support to final claims. These premises include calculations of hazard rates, confidence intervals, effect size, and $p$ values. Statistical premises like these are often theorized as objective and impersonal. However, by shifting the analytic gaze off of what, exactly, the problem is (e.g., expertise) and onto from where the problem comes (e.g., backstage material machinations), my analyses suggest that assessment conundrums persist because of the making-power of statistical methods, or their capacity and culpability in evidential attunement. Deliberators are fully aware that their method for evidential assessment provides the material-discursive parameters for detecting (or failing to detect) an effect.

Using rhetorical theory as an analytic lens allows for a re-seeing of inferential statistics' suasive properties. That is, probability might be characterized as *poesis*, and inferential statistics, specifically, can be said to include a chain of suasive enthymematic premises. Each statistical premise described above—hazard rates, confidence intervals, effect size, and $p$ values—make it possible to perform evidential assessments even when deliberators are limited to small patient samples but are expected to make generalizable claims about larger populations. In turn, each enthymematic contributor attunes deliberators to see, and thereby value, some data over others.

This chapter provides only some answers to the question about from where the problem comes during policy-making and pharmaceutical/medical deliberations. If nothing else, though, readers have witnessed that probabilistic assessments and inferential statistics are not objective and value-free tools for reporting absolute realities. Perhaps if an argument about inferential statistics as rhetoric resonated with expert deliberators, we might be able to negotiate multiple methods or ontologies (Mol 2002) by which evidences can be made to mean. Simmons and Grabill (2007) argue that "nonexpert citizens can be effective, but in order to be effective, they must have an art that is powerfully inventive and performative" (422). Two powerfully inventive and performative ways patients' cancer care and disease experiences might be accounted for in evidential assessments are through quality-of-life (QoL) questionnaires and patient-reported outcomes (or PROs).

For Fallowfield and Fleissig (2012), clinical research fails to account for the patient values and expectations to which I alluded earlier in this chapter: "The measurement of PROs, values and expectations in this setting are crucial elements that are rarely captured adequately in clinical research" (42). They go on to argue that, "despite calls for many years for inclusion of QoL variables in clinical trials, few of these latter end points are routinely measured, making it difficult to establish the real worth of new treatments. The dearth of really good quality PROs rather than clinician-reported symptoms make discussion with patients about treatment options more difficult" (Fallowfield and Fleissig 2012, 44). When competing evidences collide, as they did during the FDA's Avastin hearing, patient-reported outcomes ought not be considered tangential. They matter. Ziliak and McCloskey (2008) argue that, after all, *"there is no discipline-independent criterion for importance, calculable from the numbers alone.* Read that again. *There is no discipline-independent criterion for importance, calculable from the numbers alone.* Scientific judgment is scientific judgment, a human matter of the community of scientists. As vital as the statistical calculations are as an input into the judgment, the judgment cannot be made entirely by the statistical machinery" (168; italics in the original). Moreover, according to Fallowfield and Fleissig (2012), "even if PROs are measured they are often reported separately or incompletely" (44). They argue that biomedicine must find methods for better integrating these forms of evidence alongside or within the kinds and forms of evidence that Kaplan-Meier survival curves, for example, propose. If "more imaginative methods for analyzing and integrating PROs are required" (Fallowfield and Fleissig 2012, 44), how might technical communicators and rhetoricians assist medical professionals with developing rigorous methods for detecting, assessing, and presenting evidences that resist quantification (e.g., patient-reported outcomes and quality-of-life measures)?

In his analysis of Darwin's use of mathematics as rhetoric Wynn ([2009], drawing on Knorr Cetina's [2009] discussion of "epistemic communities," or "cultures that create and warrant knowledge" [1]) makes a case for focusing on mathematical warrants as rhetorically powerful. According to Wynn (2009), an epistemic community's commitment to a warrant determines the degree to which an argument will succeed or fail (110). Wynn distinguishes between common and special warrants in this way: common warrants "are neither challenged nor preemptively defended in an argument," while special warrants are "authorizing principles or lines of argument that are challenged when used, or require preemptive defense" (110–11). In the Avastin hearing, survival data—which, as we saw earlier, are represented visually—inhabit elite, common warrant status, while arguments characterized as "anecdotal" are substantiated by special warrants, warrants wherein "the support of further data" (Wynn 2009, 111) is either absent or missing. Recall that Aristotle describes ethos as the "default appeal, the one we rely on when others are insufficient or unavailable" (quoted in Miller 2003, 167). How, then, might technical communicators and rhetoricians help amplify the ethos of special warrants?

Inventing methods of assessment so that they are attuned to many kinds and forms of evidence—that is, both common and special warrants—without losing their methodical, disciplining ethos is desirable. If probability is *poesis* and inferential statistics is enthymematic, the rhetorical nature of evidence, therefore, ought not limit its suasive value. That Crystal and Priscilla relied on unquantifiable evidence—what some might call "mere rhetoric"—to make their case should not discount the value of that evidence. What is needed are more rigorous and transparent methods by which Crystal's and Priscilla's chains of premises, material conditions, and unquantifiable ambient rhetorics can be assessed and made to intra-act with other data.

Dr. Gawande (2014) asserts that, "in medicine and society, we have failed to recognize that people have priorities that they need us to serve besides just living longer ... the best way to learn those priorities is to ask about them" (n.p.). To their credit, concern about how to attend to patients' priorities also surfaced during the Avastin hearing:

> We would like to have better quality of life measurement tools for symptom reduction and also prevention of symptoms because these are the things that we are tasked with doing for our patients. If we can't necessarily improve survival, or even if we can, preventing symptoms, reducing symptoms, our tools just don't seem to be where they need to be although, frankly, we need greater emphasis on that.... But I just don't think our measurement tools, truthfully, for first-line metastatic breast cancer with regard to clinical benefit, are as well-established as we would like. (Avastin hearing transcripts, June 29, 2011, 161)

This quote indicates a cursory acknowledgment on the part of medical professionals that their tools for measuring and assessing evidences are not refined enough to be sensitive and responsive to patient priorities beyond "just living longer" (Gawande 2014, n.p.). Drawing on Dourish (2004), Rickert (2013) argues, "We should not understand information as decontextualized ... we should begin to see the environment not simply as the location where information shows up or as the backdrop where human cognitive activity plays out but as an ensemble of material elements bearing up, making possible, and continually incorporated in the conducting of human activity, which is to say, a stitchwork of material, practical, and discursive relations by which any work at all can be conducted" (93). Taking to be true that probability is *poesis* and inferential statistical analysis is enthymematic, technical communicators and rhetoricians are uniquely positioned to partner with scientific deliberators as they design methodical, evidential attunements that attend to "stitchwork[s] of material, practical, and discursive relations" (Rickert 2013, 93). Partnerships between both humans and statistical methods, and scientists and (post)humanists, may enrich biomedicine's attunements to bodies in flux and facilitate the coexistence of multiple ontologies in cancer care.[16]

Flattening rhetorical events such as pharmaceutical hearings into discursive battlefields limits rhetoric to little more than a symbolic art. So in addition to identifying ways that methods of evidential attunement — specifically, inferential statistics — "bring the world into rhetorical performance" (Rickert 2013, xviii), this chapter also characterizes rhetoric as both epistemological and ontological; rhetoric does double duty by not only persuading interlocutors of the value of a certain evidential truth or reality, but also attuning them to see such evidential truths or realities in the laboratory, in the first place.

# 4. SYNTHESIZING EVIDENCE

*Infrastructure is a potent topic for ethnographic investigation,*
*encompassing the processes by which infrastructure standards are developed*
*and deployed, the dynamics of infrastructure development and maintenance,*
*the constraints that infrastructures impose, and the forms of erasure and*
*homogenization in which they engage.*
Paul Dourish and Genevieve Bell, *Divining a Digital Future*

Medical professionals are inundated constantly with data about both novel interventions and revisions to outdated therapies. Between 1993 and 2001 alone, results from approximately 200,000 randomized controlled trials were published in MEDLINE, the largest index of biomedical literature (Druss and Marcus 2005). The difficulty that medical professionals experience when trying to keep up with the emergence of new evidence can cause life-threatening gaps between medical research and clinical practice.[1] One strategy the medical community uses to facilitate the flow and adoption of cutting-edge medical research is to create small teams of medical professionals who take responsibility for aggregating new clinical trial data, systematically assessing them and summarizing their findings in a standardized, written genre called the Cochrane Systematic Review (CSR). The Cochrane Collaboration defines Cochrane Systematic Reviews as "systematic assessments of evidence of the effects of healthcare interventions, intended to help people to make informed decisions about health care, their own or someone else's. Cochrane Reviews are needed to help ensure that healthcare decisions throughout the world can be informed by high quality, timely research evidence."

Readers are not likely to have heard of a CSR before. But the questions motivating CSRs are ones we ask every day. A wide range of medical uncertainties motivates CSR authors, including, for example: Will taking vitamin C help me stave off a cold? Does acupuncture help relieve pain from tension headaches? Do vaccines really prevent influenza? Does St. John's Wort help with depression? These are only some of the questions that authors of CSRs investigate, abstracts for which are free and available to the general public on the Cochrane website (Cochrane.org). Evidential syntheses, or CSRs, for each of these questions are apt examples of how written genres are "a frequently traveled path or way of getting symbolic action done either by an individual social actor or group of actors" (Schryer 1993, 207). Cochrane Systematic

Reviews are far from mere summaries of previously published data. They are hard-fought arguments. To examine more closely how Cochrane reviewers craft such arguments, I set out to study the backstage, material-discursive labor involved in synthesizing cancer-related clinical trial data into CSRs.[2]

One of the reasons why keeping up with cancer-related clinical trial data is so difficult is because just as cancer cells replicate and spread uncontrollably, so, too, do technologies and techniques used to detect and intervene on these cells. For example, in the last two decades alone, medical standards for treating breast cancer have changed more than sixty times. One of the better-known standards of breast cancer care that has evolved considerably over the last two decades is the bilateral mastectomy. Until very recently, many women in the earliest stages of breast cancer elected to undergo bilateral mastectomies—an extremely invasive medical intervention that involves the surgical removal of both breasts. Motivated by concerns of financial cost, body image, and loss of sexual function, Kurian et al. (2014) sought to evaluate whether bilateral mastectomies could be statistically associated with lower rates of mortality. Recently published in the *Journal of the American Medical Association*, Kurian et al.'s (2014) study compared rates of cancer reoccurrence and mortality among women who underwent bilateral mastectomies versus women who chose to undergo other, less invasive surgical interventions. The authors synthesized randomized clinical trial data from 1998 to 2011, which included 189,734 patients from the California Cancer Registry. Kurian et al. concluded that despite the fact that substantially more women were choosing to undergo bilateral mastectomies than ever before, when compared to breast-conserving surgery plus radiation, this aggressive surgical intervention was not, in fact, associated with lower mortality rates.

For women who have been diagnosed recently with breast cancer, Kurian et al.'s (2014) findings are hugely significant—but so is how the authors arrived at them. In particular, it is noteworthy that not all of the clinical trial data available to Kurian et al. were included in their synthesis. Many clinical trial results simply did not make the cut. Later in this chapter, readers will learn that some CSR authors incorporate fewer than 50 percent of the currently available evidence on a particular intervention. So how do authors charged with the task of synthesizing massive amounts of clinical trial data make choices about which evidences will or will not count in their final arguments? On what grounds do they make those decisions? To explore these questions and the rich rhetorical complexity of evidential synthesis in general, this chapter describes the argumentative labor associated with making evidential "cuts" (cf. Barad 2007, 115) when synthesizing clinical trial data. One of the fundamental assumptions motivating this chapter's study is that cuts are *"enacted* rather than *inherent"* (Barad 2007, 142; italics mine). Making evidential cuts are a tactic for evidencing a body in flux. Making evidential cuts is one method for navigating medical indeterminacy.[3]

### THE CASE OF THE COCHRANE SYSTEMATIC REVIEW

Cochrane Systematic Reviews are the result of a complex composing process. By way of example, consider McGovern et al.'s (2008) systematic review of the best way to treat pediatric obesity. To arrive at a final, published review, writers first articulate a reviewable question. Based on this guiding question, reviewers conduct searches for studies about the efficacy of nonsurgical interventions for treating childhood obesity. As a guide for deciding which studies will or will not be included in their corpus, McGovern et al. rely on criteria sanctioned by the Cochrane Collaboration—a global and independent network of experts in both medicine and methodology. After finalizing their search, reviewers begin composing their CSR. To do this, McGovern et al. must first decide which data from their study search results are relevant. Data extraction is, once again, guided by criteria outlined by the Cochrane Collaboration. From there, reviewers are charged with the task of evaluating the evidential quality of individual studies. Such a process also requires McGovern et al. to assess any potential biases that may have affected clinical trial researchers' findings. Only after all of this preparatory labor is completed can Cochrane reviewers begin the act of comparing evidence across studies. Results from such comparisons are based on the strength of the available evidence. Here again, McGovern et al. must rely on criteria set forth by the Cochrane Collaboration when determining the evidential strength of individual studies. Based on such determinations, reviewers draw conclusions about an intervention's effectiveness and safety. While the CSR genre may appear at the outset to be mere translation or summary of extant research about effective medical interventions, it embodies a rich set of procedures guided by a host of material-discursive infrastructures that guide claim making. Often, reviewers' final claims yield plain language summaries and decision aids that medical professionals can use when working with patients and their families toward some health-care decision-making end.

Note in the example above how frequently the Cochrane Collaboration intervenes discursively in the systematic review process. Who, or what, then, is the Cochrane Collaboration? According to its website, the Cochrane Collaboration is an "international, non-profit, independent organization" that ensures "information about the effects of healthcare interventions" is not only current but also "readily available worldwide." There are more than thirty-one thousand reviewers from over a hundred countries working within the collaboration. The Cochrane Collaboration "produces and disseminates systematic reviews of healthcare interventions, and promotes the search for evidence in the form of clinical trials and other studies of the effects of interventions." The emphasis that the Cochrane Collaboration places on rigor, reviewability, replicability, and evidential superiority shapes the practice of evidential synthesis.

According to a timeline posted on the Cochrane Collaboration's website, several important publications and events helped pave the way for what evidential synthesis looks like today. Key publications include Archie Cochrane's (1972) *Effectiveness and Efficiency: Random Reflections on Health Services*, which initiated the use of systematic reviews in the United Kingdom and later in the World Health Organization. In these early reviews, evidence was collected from controlled trials in perinatal medicine. Later, in 1979, Cochrane published an essay in which he argued that it was "surely a great criticism of our profession that we have not organised a critical summary, by specialty or subspecialty, adapted periodically, of all relevant randomised controlled trials" (Cochrane Community 2013). Soon after, international collaborations developed to conduct systematic reviews of controlled trials in pregnancy, childbirth, and the neonatal period.

In the early 1990s, Michael Peckham (the first director of research and development in the British National Health Service) approved funding for a Cochrane Centre to "facilitate the preparation of systematic reviews of randomised controlled trials of health care" (Cochrane Community 2013). A team of medical professionals, including Gordon Guyatt (whose definition of evidence-based medicine is cited quite frequently), met at McMaster University in Hamilton, Ontario, Canada, to develop principles for the Cochrane Centre. That same year (1992), the Cochrane Centre opened. The Cochrane Centre developed and organized review groups focused on medical specialties (e.g., strokes, pregnancy and childbirth).

In addition to human expertise, the Cochrane Centre learned how to leverage the affordances of computational labor. In 1994, they deployed the first version of "RevMan"—a software system that managed writers' reviews. A database of systematic reviews (designed by Update Software) was also rolled out. Because of the large-scale nature of the Cochrane Collaboration's project and its technological sophistication, comparisons to the Human Genome Project emerged. In 1995, an article in the *Lancet* suggested that the Cochrane Collaboration was "an enterprise that rivals the Human Genome Project in its potential implications for modern medicine" (Bero and Rennie 1995). In 1996, the database of systematic reviews was available online, and one year later, comments and criticisms could also be made online.

The Cochrane Collaboration's reputation continues to thrive. Between 2001 and 2003, the Cochrane library went from publishing one thousand systematic reviews to more than three thousand. Having garnered the respect of the medical community by convincing them of the importance of rigorous and systematic reviews, in 2005, the *Lancet* began to require authors who submit manuscripts to include a "clear summary of previous research findings, ideally by direct reference to a systematic review" (Chalmers et al. 2014). In 2011, the Cochrane Collaboration was accepted as a nongovernmental organization in official relations with the World Health Organization, and by 2012 the number of reviews in the Cochrane database exceeded five thousand. To date, the Cochrane Collaboration has turned its investigative gaze toward qualitative studies.

Contemporary evidence-based medicine's emergence runs parallel to the medical community's adoption of the CSR genre. In interviews with a panel of medical professionals who spearheaded the evidence-based medicine movement, Gordon Guyatt indicated that the root of the CSR is evidence-based medicine and that the predecessor to CSRs were what he called "critical appraisals." Critical appraisals were meta-analyses of all available evidence. Meta-analysis, according to participants on the evidence-based medicine panel, "is a logical way of dealing with the medical literature ... and dealing with a practical patient problem" (Chalmers et al. 2014). Another participant in the panel, Brian Haynes, stated that he often wondered "how much of my medical training ... had been based on theories that were not supported by facts?" (Chalmers et al. 2014). When asked to articulate what evidence-based medicine does that critical appraisals do not, David L. Sackett argued that evidence-based medicine goes beyond critical appraisals in that they integrate the science and literature with best clinical skills. Sackett claims, "Help versus harm is determined using patient values ... patients can then weigh the two possible outcomes" (Chalmers et al., 2014). All panelists described that prior to evidence-based medicine's ability to assert an intervention's efficacy based on statistical analyses, medical authority and expertise were limited to confident articulations of anecdotal evidence and previous clinical experiences.

Cochrane Systematic Reviews are not foolproof, however. First, they have limited application for patients with comorbidities (or more than one illness). In other words, CSRs might only attend to a fraction of a patient's corporeal concerns. When medical scientists conduct the actual clinical trial, comorbidities can complicate a researcher's capacity to isolate and distinguish between an intervention's effects and the results of a complicated disease profile (or some combination thereof). Second, many clinical trials that, ideally, could or should have been incorporated into a CSR never see the light of day. There are a number of reasons why clinical trials are not published, including the reality that, over time, some researchers simply become uninterested in the study, while others may lose funding for the research. Third, publication bias limits how comprehensive, inclusive, and accurate reviewers' whole-scale assessments of extant research can be. Despite these and other limitations, Ian Chalmers insists that "we need to find out what we know already. We haven't gotten anywhere near that yet." For Chalmers, CSRs are integral to medical practice because they unearth and summarize care solutions that medical professionals may be unaware of or unconvinced by.

The iterative process of aggregating and assessing multiple evidences from many sources and then making evidential cuts is perhaps one of the most important and time-consuming aspects of medical professionals' practice. The act of composing a CSR relies on intra-actions between humans, heuristics, and software in the search for and sifting of evidence. Findings from CSRs have the authority to change clinical practitioners' minds and the power to improve patients' prognoses. Unlike other groups of experts that convene to build standards through evidential examinations, the Cochrane Foundation boasts financial isolation from pharmaceutical companies. It stands to reason, then, that arguments within CSRs are unaffected by outside financial interests.

According to informal conversations with a regular CSR reviewer and after analyzing documents designed by the Cochrane Collaboration to guide the review process, the following prepublication practices summarize reviewer activity.

*Planning*
Reviewers compose a protocol and submit it to the Cochrane Collaboration. The Cochrane Collaboration reviews the protocol and, in most cases, asks for revisions. To write the protocol, reviewers rely on the *Cochrane Handbook* (Higgins and Green 2011), which includes a checklist referred to as PRISMA, or "preferred reporting items for systematic reviews and meta-analyses" (see fig. 4.1).

*Searching*
Reviewers conduct either (and in some cases, both) electronic and/or hand searches for articles. Many reviewers are indebted to medical librarians for the immense amount of search support they provide to reviewers.

**PRISMA 2009 Checklist**

| Section/topic | # | Checklist item | Reported on page # |
|---|---|---|---|
| **TITLE** | | | |
| Title | 1 | Identify the report as a systematic review, meta-analysis, or both. | |
| **ABSTRACT** | | | |
| Structured summary | 2 | Provide a structured summary including, as applicable: background; objectives; data sources; study eligibility criteria, participants, and interventions; study appraisal and synthesis methods; results; limitations; conclusions and implications of key findings; systematic review registration number. | |
| **INTRODUCTION** | | | |
| Rationale | 3 | Describe the rationale for the review in the context of what is already known. | |
| Objectives | 4 | Provide an explicit statement of questions being addressed with reference to participants, interventions, comparisons, outcomes, and study design (PICOS). | |
| **METHODS** | | | |
| Protocol and registration | 5 | Indicate if a review protocol exists, if and where it can be accessed (e.g., Web address), and, if available, provide registration information including registration number. | |
| Eligibility criteria | 6 | Specify study characteristics (e.g., PICOS, length of follow-up) and report characteristics (e.g., years considered, language, publication status) used as criteria for eligibility, giving rationale. | |
| Information sources | 7 | Describe all information sources (e.g., databases with dates of coverage, contact with study authors to identify additional studies) in the search and date last searched. | |
| Search | 8 | Present full electronic search strategy for at least one database, including any limits used, such that it could be repeated. | |
| Study selection | 9 | State the process for selecting studies (i.e., screening, eligibility, included in systematic review, and, if applicable, included in the meta-analysis). | |
| Data collection process | 10 | Describe method of data extraction from reports (e.g., piloted forms, independently, in duplicate) and any processes for obtaining and confirming data from investigators. | |
| Data items | 11 | List and define all variables for which data were sought (e.g., PICOS, funding sources) and any assumptions and simplifications made. | |
| Risk of bias in individual studies | 12 | Describe methods used for assessing risk of bias of individual studies (including specification of whether this was done at the study or outcome level), and how this information is to be used in any data synthesis. | |
| Summary measures | 13 | State the principal summary measures (e.g., risk ratio, difference in means). | |
| Synthesis of results | 14 | Describe the methods of handling data and combining results of studies, if done, including measures of consistency (e.g., $I^2$) for each meta-analysis. | |

 **PRISMA 2009 Checklist**

| Section/topic | # | Checklist item | Reported on page # |
|---|---|---|---|
| Risk of bias across studies | 15 | Specify any assessment of risk of bias that may affect the cumulative evidence (e.g., publication bias, selective reporting within studies). | |
| Additional analyses | 16 | Describe methods of additional analyses (e.g., sensitivity or subgroup analyses, meta-regression), if done, indicating which were pre-specified. | |
| **RESULTS** | | | |
| Study selection | 17 | Give numbers of studies screened, assessed for eligibility, and included in the review, with reasons for exclusions at each stage, ideally with a flow diagram. | |
| Study characteristics | 18 | For each study, present characteristics for which data were extracted (e.g., study size, PICOS, follow-up period) and provide the citations. | |
| Risk of bias within studies | 19 | Present data on risk of bias of each study and, if available, any outcome level assessment (see item 12). | |
| Results of individual studies | 20 | For all outcomes considered (benefits or harms), present, for each study: (a) simple summary data for each intervention group (b) effect estimates and confidence intervals, ideally with a forest plot. | |
| Synthesis of results | 21 | Present results of each meta-analysis done, including confidence intervals and measures of consistency. | |
| Risk of bias across studies | 22 | Present results of any assessment of risk of bias across studies (see Item 15). | |
| Additional analysis | 23 | Give results of additional analyses, if done (e.g., sensitivity or subgroup analyses, meta-regression [see Item 16]). | |
| **DISCUSSION** | | | |
| Summary of evidence | 24 | Summarize the main findings including the strength of evidence for each main outcome; consider their relevance to key groups (e.g., healthcare providers, users, and policy makers). | |
| Limitations | 25 | Discuss limitations at study and outcome level (e.g., risk of bias), and at review-level (e.g., incomplete retrieval of identified research, reporting bias). | |
| Conclusions | 26 | Provide a general interpretation of the results in the context of other evidence, and implications for future research. | |
| **FUNDING** | | | |
| Funding | 27 | Describe sources of funding for the systematic review and other support (e.g., supply of data); role of funders for the systematic review. | |

*From:* Moher D, Liberati A, Tetzlaff J, Altman DG, The PRISMA Group (2009). Preferred Reporting Items for Systematic Reviews and Meta-Analyses: The PRISMA Statement. PLoS Med 6(7): e1000097. doi:10.1371/journal.pmed1000097

For more information, visit: www.prisma-statement.org.

Figure 4.1 PRISMA checklist, pages 1 and 2

### Consensus

In some cases, review teams have a coordinator who develops a document (sometimes using PowerPoint) that summarizes research questions and relevant, useful articles located during the search process. After circulating this document to team members, he or she will solicit feedback and ask questions such as:

- What did we find here?
- Does what we found correspond to our research question?
- What's the "so-what" of what we found?

Once consensus is reached on answers to these and other CSR-specific questions, reviewers extract relevant data and enter them into Archie, an online repository for CSR documents and other data about review teams' contact information. According to the Archie website (http://tech.cochrane.org /archie), within Archie it is possible to read, print, and compare current and past versions of a document.

### Material Composing

Using the PRISMA checklist as a heuristic, reviewers begin composing their written review of available evidence. Within Archie, reviewers use RevMan (short for "review manager") to prepare and maintain their reviews. According to the Archie website, reviewers can use RevMan for both protocols and full reviews. Moreover, RevMan, "is most useful when you have formulated the question for the review, and allows you to prepare the text, build the tables showing the characteristics of studies and the comparisons in the review, and add study data. It can perform meta-analyses and present the results graphically" (http://tech.cochrane.org/revman). One reviewer stated that the Cochrane Collaboration's guidelines make this process pretty black and white and that the act itself is akin to "filling in the blanks." When prompted for specifics about how she knows how to materially compose the review, she replied that she "just does what Archie wants her to do."

In most cases, the first draft of the CSR is composed by the team coordinator and then circulated to the team for feedback. Occasionally, drafts are written right in Archie since one of its technological affordances is that it maintains the integrity of the sorting and search process. Since it is so central to the act of sorting and ranking evidence, the PRISMA checklist may be placed in a visible location while composing the written review. Although the editorial process workflow diagram is provided (see fig. 4.2 for one example from the Acute Respiratory Infections Cochrane group), teams are not wedded to this order of operations. Reviewers appraise the quality of evidence using

**ARI COCHRANE REVIEW GROUP – FLOW DIAGRAM OF EDITORIAL PROCESSES**

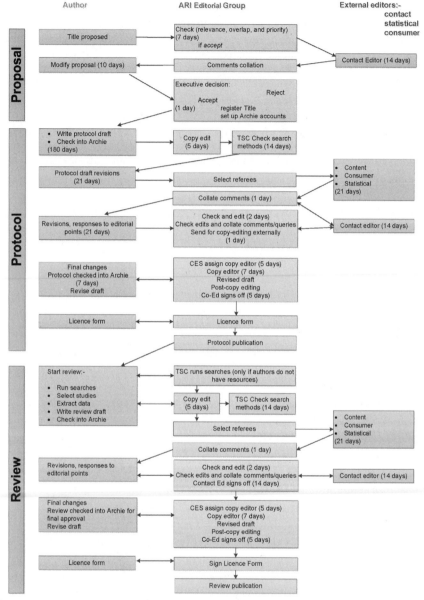

Figure 4.2 Cochrane's Acute Respiratory Infections Group:
editorial process diagram (source: http://ari.cochrane.org/sites/ari
.cochrane.org/files/uploads/Editorial%20Process.pdf)

| Underlying methodology | Quality rating |
|---|---|
| Randomized trials; or double-upgraded observational studies. | High |
| Downgraded randomized trials; or upgraded observational studies. | Moderate |
| Double-downgraded randomized trials; or observational studies. | Low |
| Triple-downgraded randomized trials; or downgraded observational studies; or case series/case reports. | Very low |

Figure 4.3 GRADE criteria (source: Higgins and Green 2011, table 12.2)

GRADE criteria (fig. 4.3), which stands for "grading of recommendations assessment, development and evaluation." These criteria allow appraisals to be presented alongside confidence intervals. (See chap. 3 in this book for an in-depth examination of statistical analysis, including confidence intervals, as yet another method for making evidential cuts in medical practice.)

In addition to the four workflow stages preceding publication of the review (fig. 4.2), there is an official publication process whereby journal editors may require that the manuscript be submitted with a PRISMA checklist as well as an articulation of the review's potential impact. Once the review is published, original authors take responsibility for updating or revising the review every two years in light of additional evidence (although, in some cases, teams may inherit an update). The Cochrane Collaboration grants preapprovals of all protocols and all subsequent revisions.

Finally, to disseminate CSR findings widely, reviewers' data are translated into plain language summaries. Medical professionals may later incorporate these plain language summaries into patient decision aids, which requires translating and interpreting for nonexpert readers not just a CSR's statistical evidence but also the validity of reviewers' findings. To do this, writers rely on GRADE criteria, which allow authors to communicate such information through probabilities. Now that I have outlined the generalizable process by which CSRs as a genre come to be, I analyze, in what follows, the backstage, rhetorical labor involved in crafting individual CSRs.

### EVIDENTIAL SYNTHESES AS RHETORIC

I will now shed light on the material-discursive labor involved in making evidential cuts and thereby contribute to ongoing conversations about the rhetorical nature of standards. The fundamental assumption guiding this analysis is that examining standards in formation and standards' information (Oyama et al. 2000, 12) poses the power to demonstrate how data ultimately become actionable. Forthcoming models for how medical professionals synthesize evidences to craft arguments about treatment options may offer help-

**Table 4.1 Cancer, Exigency, and CSR Citation**

| Cancer | Exigency | CSR |
|---|---|---|
| Lung | Most common form of cancer; cause of most cancer-related deaths worldwide. (Ferlay et al. 2015) | Manser et al. 2013 |
| Prostate | Second most prevalent cancer and sixth leading cause of death in men worldwide. Most commonly diagnosed cancer in developed countries and third leading cause of death in men in those countries. (Jemal 2011) | Ilic et al. 2013 |
| Breast | Most common cancer in women worldwide. (Ferlay et al. 2015) | Gøtzsche and Jørgensen 2013 |

ful heuristics for teaching evidence-based medicine's argumentative infrastructure.

According to the World Health Organization, in 2012, fourteen million new cancer diagnoses were made worldwide. That same year, another 8.2 million people died from cancer. The World Health Organization estimates that, when 2014 calculations are made, this number of new cancer cases will increase by about an astounding 70 percent. Motivated by these data, I conduct a rhetorical analysis of three specific CSRs about effective cancer-screening protocols. One of the top five most common cancer diagnoses among both men and women is lung cancer. For men, prostate cancer is also among the top five cancer diagnoses, while for women, breast cancer is among the top five. Based on these statistics, and to maintain the manageability of the study, I limit my analysis to CSRs that review the efficacy of cancer screening for lung cancer, breast cancer, and prostate cancer (see table 4.1). Specifically, I analyze Manser et al.'s (2013) "Screening for Lung Cancer (Review)," Ilic et al.'s (2013) "Screening for Prostate Cancer (Review)," and Gøtzsche and Jørgensen's (2013) "Screening for Breast Cancer with Mammography (Review)." Each rhetorical analysis allows for one peek behind the scenes at how evidences that will one day become argumentative grounds on which decisions are made come to be.

For each of the three aforementioned CSRs I, (1) map their textual features, (2) trace reviewers' review activity (as can be deduced from reviewers' descriptions within the CSR), and (3) conduct rhetorical analyses of their extratextual features.[4] I mobilize both Toulmin's model for argumentation and stasis theory as an analytic lens for identifying moments when (and why) evidential cuts are made.

## The Textual Features of CSRs

Each of the three CSRs adheres to a stable set of typified genre conventions, resulting in a list of rather consistent textual features. After providing introductory details and an abstract for readers, every review begins with background information followed by a brief and explicit description of reviewers' objectives. Each CSR then describes in great detail reviewers' methods for conducting the review. Frequently, reviewers reference key charter documents that guided the review process, including various editions of the CSR Handbook (Higgins and Green 2005, 2008, 2011) and key publications outlining the criteria reviewers used to assess evidence (Guyatt et al. 2008, 2011). After describing their methods, reviewers go on to present results. These results include (*a*) a description of which studies were included, (*b*) a methodological critique of each study included in the review, and (*c*) statistical analyses of individual and pooled effects for each cancer-screening approach. Reviewers then summarize their results and comment on the quality of evidence in the original studies. They also attend to any potential methodological biases they were unable to avoid in their review (e.g., encountering missing data). When applicable, reviewers acknowledge distinctions between this review and previous reviews of the same cancer-screening practices. Finally, each of the three CSRs makes an argument about practical implications for both clinical practice and future research.

After the formal review ends, what follows are a series of tables and figures provided in the CSR's appendices. Appendices include visual and statistical illustrations along with textual detail about each of the review's findings. Figures and tables report on pooled data analyses from studies that make a case for a specific cancer-screening protocol. In this section of the CSR, readers are provided greater detail about statistical differences between studies' control treatment arms. Importantly, in both the appendices and the body of the CSR, reviewers provide detailed descriptions about how they managed the complex task of deciding which studies would be included and which studies would have to be excluded from their syntheses. More often than not, Cochran reviewers cite as justification for cutting a study from their synthesis the fact that the original study's methodology was weak or biased in some way. Reviewers also describe how they harnessed and homogenized data for the sake of comparison. As I'll describe in greater detail, these two rhetorical moves—excluding and homogenizing data—are central to the task of conducting evidential syntheses.

Finally, each review includes back matter that describes electronic database search strategies, what's new about this review compared with previous reviews, the history of the investigation (i.e., when the last time this review was updated), authorial contributions, declarations of interest, sources of support, any differences between the protocol originally proposed to Cochrane versus what was finally published, and index terms. Figure 4.4 provides a (rather overwhelming) visual illustration of the argumentative anatomy and concomitant textual features of CSRs. Specifically, figure 4.4 highlights the six main textual components of CSRs: review objectives, background, methods, results, discussion, and conclusions. Figure 4.4 also demonstrates the rhetorical moves and evidence that help buttress each of those six sections. For example, in the methods section of CSRs, reviewers indicate their criteria for inclusion, methods they used to find relevant clinical trials, and details about how they collected and analyzed data. Figure 4.4 drills down even further by indicating the specific criteria reviewers use to include and exclude evidences: types of outcome measures (which may be primary and/or secondary outcomes), types of studies, types of participants, and types of interventions. With regard to search methods, figure 4.4 illustrates that electronic database searches are the primary method—details of which are always provided in the appendices of the reviews. And finally, when reviewers attend to methods for data collection and analysis, they answer the following questions in the methods sections: How did we select studies? And for each of those studies, how did we extract and manage data, assess bias, measure treatment effects, deal with missing data, assess heterogeneity, synthesize data using RevMan and the random-effects model, conduct subgroup analyses, and conduct sensitivity analyses? Figure 4.4 serves as an illustration of the argumentative anatomy and the relationships between different levels of evidence-based argumentation in CSRs.

## Reviewers' Activity

For each of the three CSRs, I identified every action verb that reviewers used when describing a particular activity they performed (see table 4.2). The decision to locate action verbs as a way to account for reviewer activity was made, in part, because during this project's exploratory study, it was clear that reviewers relied on a rather stable and routine set of procedures. Their stability, I hypothesize, makes it possible to identify when systematic reviewers perform evidential cutting.

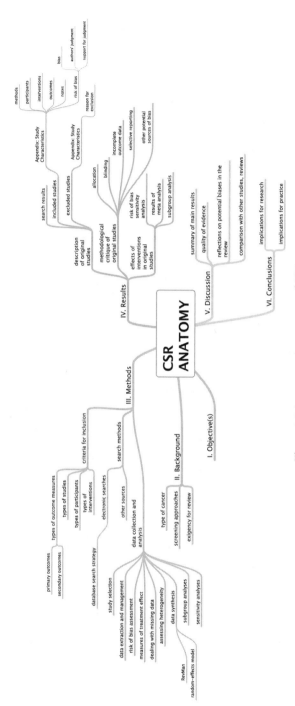

Figure 4.4 Argumentative anatomy of CSRs

**Table 4.2 CSR Reviewer Activity**

| Step | Manser, Lethaby, Irving, Stone, Byrnes, Abramson, and Campbell (2013): "Screening for Lung Cancer" | Ilic, Neuberger, Djulbegovic, and Dahm (2013): "Screening for Prostate Cancer" | Gøtzsche and Jørgensen (2013): "Screening for Breast Cancer with Mammography" |
|---|---|---|---|
| 1 | Determined inclusion/exclusion criteria | Determined eligibility for included studies | Determined inclusion/exclusion criteria |
| 2 | Determined which outcomes would be measured | Determined eligibility of participants for included studies | Searched PubMed using specific search terms |
| 3 | Determined search methods | Determined what kinds of screening procedures would be included | Searched WHO's International Clinical Trials Registry Platform using specific search strategies |
| 4 | Hand searched the journal *Lung Cancer*, 1985–2000, including abstracts from international lung cancer meetings | Determined what outcomes would be measured (both primary and secondary outcomes) | Scanned reference lists |
| 5 | Searched bibliographies of identified studies for additional citations | Conducted electronic and manual searches (search strategy is detailed in Ilic et al., app. 1) | Included letters, abstracts, grey literature, unpublished data |
| 6 | Searched narrative reviews for additional citations | Hand searched reviews, technical reviews, and gray literature | Independently decided which trials to include based on prestated criteria |

**Table 4.2 Continued**

| Step | Manser, Lethaby, Irving, Stone, Byrnes, Abramson, and Campbell (2013): "Screening for Lung Cancer" | Ilic, Neuberger, Djulbegovic, and Dahm (2013): "Screening for Prostate Cancer" | Gøtzsche and Jørgensen (2013): "Screening for Breast Cancer with Mammography" |
|---|---|---|---|
| 7 | Contacted authors of primary studies and experts in the field of lung cancer screening to ask whether they were aware of any additional relevant unpublished or published studies or works in progress | Contacted authors of studies included in review | Resolved disagreements by discussion |
| 8 | Searched titles and abstracts for potentially relevant trials for full review obtained from initial electronic search | Manually searched abstracts from three meetings (American Urological Association, European Association of Urology, American Society of Clinical Oncology) | Assessed randomization adequacy (using Higgins and Green 2008) |
| 9 | Determined which studies would be included/excluded | Used Higgins and Green 2011 (*Cochrane Handbook*) as guide for collecting and analyzing data | Divided trials into those with adequate randomization vs. those with suboptimal randomization |
| 10 | Assessed full texts of retrieved studies to determine if they met inclusion criteria | Independently selected trials against a predetermined checklist of inclusion criteria: (*a*) Categorized studies into one of two groups: possibly relevant; excluded; and (*b*) Resolved discrepancies between authors via discussion | Extracted methodological and outcome data |

*Synthesizing Evidence*

**Table 4.2 Continued**

| Step | Manser, Lethaby, Irving, Stone, Byrnes, Abramson, and Campbell (2013): "Screening for Lung Cancer" | Ilic, Neuberger, Djulbegovic, and Dahm (2013): "Screening for Prostate Cancer" | Gøtzsche and Jørgensen (2013): "Screening for Breast Cancer with Mammography" |
|---|---|---|---|
| 11 | Measured agreement using simple consensus and kappa statistics | Independently extracted data using standard data extraction form, resolved discrepancies by consensus | Resolved disagreements by discussion |
| 12 | Resolved disagreement by adjudication of a third party or by consensus | Data extraction form was pilot tested and modified before using | Contacted primary investigators to clarify uncertainties |
| 13 | Assessed biases (using *Cochrane Handbook*; used as measures "low/ unclear/high" bias) | Recorded quality charac-teristics of trial | Performed intention-to-treat analyses |
| 14 | Measured interauthor reliability using kappa and weighted kappa statistics | Recorded results of trial | Used fixed-effect model with Mantel-Haenszel method |
| 15 | Extracted data and entered into them into RevMan | Recorded participant details | When heterogeneous ($p < .10$), explored possible causes |
| 16 | Extrapolated otherwise unavailable data from graphs | Recorded types of screening interventions used | Presented analyses in graphs as risk ratios |
| 17 | Reported risk ratios with 95% confidence intervals for dichotomous outcomes | Recorded outcomes reported, including types of measures used to record the outcome | Discussed absolute risk reductions/increases and risk differences |

**Table 4.2 Continued**

| Step | Manser, Lethaby, Irving, Stone, Byrnes, Abramson, and Campbell (2013): "Screening for Lung Cancer" | Ilic, Neuberger, Djulbegovic, and Dahm (2013): "Screening for Prostate Cancer" | Gøtzsche and Jørgensen (2013): "Screening for Breast Cancer with Mammography" |
|---|---|---|---|
| 18 | Tested homogeneity, $p < .10$ as cut-off (as per Higgins et al. 2003) | Assessed bias (low/moderate/high—per Higgins and Green 2005) in original review by reporting the trial's conduct against particular criteria | Reported outcome data at 7 and 13 years and presented age groups under 50 years and above |
| 19 | Calculated $I^2$ statistic for pooled analyses | Assessed bias in updated review (using criteria in Higgins and Green 2011) and using a question-based entry (yes = low; no = high; unclear) | ... |
| 20 | Reported risk ratios using random-effects model where there was significant statistical heterogeneity | Rated quality of evidence using GRADE (per Guyatt et al. 2011) | ... |
| 21 | Used fixed-effects model for other outcomes | Analyzed treatment effects statistically (per statistical guidelines referenced in Higgins and Green 2011) | ... |
| 22 | Analyzed data on an intention-to-screen basis | Dealt with missing data by contacting original study investigators to request missing data; when unavailable, analysis was performed on what was available | ... |

*Synthesizing Evidence*

**Table 4.2 Continued**

| Step | Manser, Lethaby, Irving, Stone, Byrnes, Abramson, and Campbell (2013): "Screening for Lung Cancer" | Ilic, Neuberger, Djulbegovic, and Dahm (2013): "Screening for Prostate Cancer" | Gøtzsche and Jørgensen (2013): "Screening for Breast Cancer with Mammography" |
|---|---|---|---|
| 23 | Assessed statistical significance of differences using Fisher's Exact test | Assessed heterogeneity using graphical interpretation of forest plot and the $I^2$ statistic (above 75% was considered considerable heterogeneity; per Higgins and Green 2011) | ... |
| 24 | Used conservative Bonferroni correction to adjust for multiple comparisons (as per Bland 1995) | Evaluated clinical heterogeneity (using patient characteristics) and screening and subsequent treatment protocols | ... |
| 25 | ... | Assessed reporting biases using forest plots | ... |
| 26 | ... | Synthesized data using random-effects model (using RevMan 2011) | ... |
| 27 | ... | Conducted subgroup analysis exploring screening of men aged greater than or equal to 45, 50, and 55 years old | ... |
| 28 | ... | Performed several post hoc sensitivity analyses | ... |

A methodological caveat: I understand that not all review activities can be accounted for by examining only reviewers' final, written descriptions of their processes. However, because the preparation and review process is so arduous, reviewers sometimes invest years of their careers to complete and update syntheses. Indeed, post hoc analyses are limiting in that they cannot reveal the informal, intermediary genres and ad hoc activities that mediate reviewers' practices (see Spinuzzi, Hart-Davidson, and Zachry's [2006] "Chains and Ecologies"). However, I hope that by tracing and analyzing reviewers' explicit references to actual review activity, readers might have a more complete sense of this labor than we do at present. I also hope that this research will help shape methods for future studies of real-time review activity.

In both the exploratory study for this project and in the analysis of the following cancer-screening CSRs, tracing reviewers' activity rendered anywhere from eighteen to twenty-eight specific practices. Following Farkas and Haas's (2012) description of grounded theory analysis as a series of iterative movements involving pushing out and pulling in, I reduced this study's open codes to seven, overarching reviewer activities. These include:

- establishing inclusion/exclusion criteria and search methods
- assessing original studies' methodological biases
- extracting data
- analyzing data statistically
- synthesizing data (except in the breast cancer–screening CSR)
- determining the quality of evidence (except in the breast cancer–screening CSR)
- performing sensitivity analyses (except in the breast cancer–screening CSR)

Because reviewers in the breast cancer–screening CSR found themselves hampered by what they described as methodological issues within the original studies, there was no explicit mention of the final three activities listed above.

After constant comparison of each of these seven general activities, and in accordance with Farkas and Haas (2012), codes were further pulled in and summarized, which resulted in the following conclusion: systematic reviewers' practices revolve around addressing two very important questions. (1) How (and how well) did we do what we did? (2) How (and how well) did they (original researchers) do what they did? Both of these questions are clearly related to concerns about (methodological) procedure. Figure 4.5 illustrates the relationship between reviewers' explicitly stated activities and these two procedural queries.

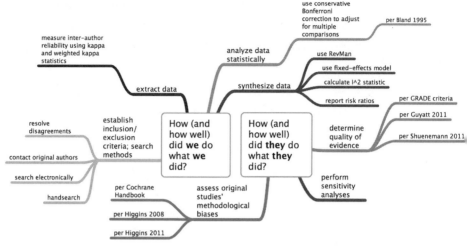

Figure 4.5 CSR reviewers' activity as related to two overarching procedural questions

With respect to the question "How (and how well) did *we* do what *we* did?" reviewers back their claims through explicit articulations of (*a*) how they resolved disagreements about inclusion and exclusion criteria, contacted authors of original studies for clarification about original studies, and conducted electronic searches; (*b*) how they extracted actual data and used kappa and weighted kappa statistics to measure inter-author agreement about those data; (*c*) how they used inferential statistics to analyze data, and, per Bland and Altman (1995), used conservative Bonferroni correction to adjust for multiple comparisons; and (*d*) how they synthesized their data using RevMan, the fixed-effects model, the $I^2$ statistic, and described risk ratios.

With respect to the question "How (and how well) did *they* do what *they* did?" reviewers (*a*) use the Cochrane Handbook (Higgins and Green 2005, 2008, 2011) to assess the methodological biases of the original studies; (*b*) perform sensitivity analyses on original studies; and (*c*) determine the quality of original studies using current GRADE criteria, Guyatt et al. (2008), and Guyatt et al. (2011).

As illustrated in figure 4.5, CSRs attempt to answer the following questions: What procedures did *we*, the reviewers use, in order to conduct our review? What methodological shortcomings, if any, did *we* encounter as *we* deployed those procedures? What procedures did *original researchers* (whose data we now employ in our own research) use? What methodological shortcomings, if any, can be located in *original researchers'* procedures? Answers to these questions fortify final claims about cancer-screening recommendations. Ultimately, these questions embody concerns about how cuts are enacted "between the object and the agencies of observation" (Barad 2007, 268).

## The Extratextual Features of CSRs: A Toulminian Analysis

At first glance, each CSR presents a series of very logical, objective reasons for why reviewers recommend a particular cancer-screening approach. This would be especially true for readers who only read abstracts and plain language summaries. Highlighting reviewers' activity helps unearth additional details about reviewers' practices. But reviewer activity can tell us only so much. A more detailed explication of reviewers' rhetorical reasoning is necessary if we're to understand how, exactly, reviewers conduct the backstage, synthesizing labor that grants documents like CSRs the authority to catalyze clinical practice. Pairing details about the anatomy of CSR arguments and reviewers' practices with theories in classical and contemporary rhetoric unveils some of reviewers' rhetorical reasoning.

In previous research, I used Toulmin's model for argumentation to understand how standard of care documents maintained their authority even as they were deployed judiciously, depending on the expertise and experience of individual medical professionals (see Teston 2009). Since standard of care documents and CSRs are similar synthesizing genres (but not necessarily parallel documents), in what follows, I extend Toulmin's model to CSRs as an analytic frame. As indicated above, all CSR activity can be traced back to two general queries about procedural concerns: (1) How (and how well) did *we* do what *we* did? (2) How (and how well) did *they* (original researchers) do what *they* did? Toulmin's model provides language for identifying how reviewers make certain argumentative moves when answering such questions. Ultimately, these argumentative moves lie at the heart of evidential synthesis.

According to Toulmin's model, there are four major elements of any argument—claims, grounds, warrants, and backing. Additionally, qualifiers indicate the strength or generalizability of the claim, and rebuttals offer up a counterargument to the claim. For Toulmin et al. (1984), claims are an argument's "destination" (25), while grounds (i.e., "common ground") support claims based on facts on which we can all agree (38). Grounds might be thought of as the reply one might give were someone to ask, "Well, what do you have to go on?" Warrants are statements that indicate how facts on which we all agree are connected (often implicitly) to the claim. It may be helpful to think of warrants as license to make a claim. Backing, according to Toulmin et al. (1984), includes generalizations that make explicit the body of experience that an interlocutor relies on to establish the trustworthiness of an argumentative method (61).

When synthesizing evidences, reviewers must deploy value-laden evidential cuts. In the ensuing Toulminian analyses, I illustrate how making these evidential cuts is akin to what Haraway (1988) might call a god trick, or an idealized form of objectivity that is impossible to achieve. In particular, to conduct a CSR, I conclude that reviewers perform the illusion of objectivity in four ways.

1. Flatten data from the original clinical trials. That is, reviewers must find ways to make heterogeneous data homogenous for the sake of comparison. Strategies for accomplishing this are typically statistical in nature (e.g., conservative Bonferroni correction, weighted kappas for inter-author reliability, sensitivity analyses, risk ratios).[5]
2. Devalue narrative as a reliable method for making sense of the world.
3. Overlook the role of relationships between humans and their environment when measuring an intervention's efficacy.
4. Ignore the role of funding sources (e.g., from pharmaceutical corporations, private donations, and government) when determining the viability and value of original studies' research questions.

In what follows, I provide the analytic details that support these findings.

## Toulminian Analysis of Lung Cancer–Screening CSR

To date, lung cancer is the number one cause of cancer-related deaths in the United States. More than two years ago, one cancer center in the United States (Adena) began to offer free CT scans for lung cancer screening. As I write this, Adena has screened 1,190 unique patients for lung cancer and, thus far, claims to have diagnosed fourteen cases of lung cancer. Additionally, Adena has identified one instance of breast cancer and multiple instances wherein patients presented with heart aneurysms and other thoracic complications that may have become life threatening at some point in the future. Adena Cancer Center is not the only institution that now covers lung cancer screening. Medicare also currently pays for lung cancer screening.

Readers might wonder what could possibly go wrong with screening for lung cancer, especially given the fact that Adena Cancer Center was able to detect other potentially life-threatening diseases. Many experts maintain that lung cancer screening not only leads to a number of false positives but also is a costly expense whose efficacy is unsupported by data. In response to such critiques, Manser et al. (2013) set out to review evidence that would determine if screening for lung cancer reduces lung cancer mortality. Results from a Toulminian analysis of this CSR can be found in table 4.3.

Manser et al.'s (2013) overarching argument (or Toulminian claim) is:

**Table 4.3 Toulminian Analysis of "Screening for Lung Cancer" (Manser et al. 2013)**

| Toulmin's Construct | Associated Argumentative Move |
|---|---|
| Claim | "Screening with annual plain chest radiography in smokers and non-smokers, and more frequent chest radiography screening in smokers and ex-smokers, is not effective at reducing lung cancer mortality and cannot be recommended for clinical practice." |
| Grounds | A statistical meta-analysis of nine trials ($n$ = 453,965) does not support screening for lung cancer. |
| Warrants | Cochrane review methods (including GRADE, PRISMA, *Cochrane Handbook*). |
| Backing | Original studies. |
| Qualifier | "More research is needed." |
| Rebuttal | Low dose annual CT screening for high-risk smokers may have a statistically significant effect on reducing mortality. |

"Screening with annual plain chest radiography in smokers and non-smokers, and more frequent chest radiography screening in smokers and ex-smokers, is not effective at reducing lung cancer mortality and cannot be recommended for clinical practice" (21). Grounds on which they base this claim include statistical meta-analyses of nine trials that, in total, included 453,965 participants. As I argued in chapter 3, inferential statistical analyses are the standard method of medical professionals for examining the efficacy and safety of interventions. This method, therefore, acts as the Toulminian "common ground" on which we can all agree. Manser et al. warrant their claim with references to several of Cochrane's standardized review methods, including GRADE, PRISMA, and the *Cochrane Handbook*. In the CSR's appendices, Manser et al. provide analyses of each individual clinical trial, including not only the nine trials they incorporated into their final review, but also a description of the other trials that they chose to exclude from their review. Analyses in Manser et al.'s appendices help to back, in a Toulminian sense, their final claim. As is the case with most CSRs, Manser et al. qualify their claim with the statement that "more research is needed" (2013, 2). The authors offer up one possible counterargument to their claim: while lung cancer screening for smokers and ex-smokers does not help to reduce lung cancer mortality rates, low-dose annual CT screening for *high-risk* smokers may, in fact, have a statistically significant effect on reducing lung cancer–related mortality.

Readers should note that while nine trials were included in Manser et al.'s (2013) CSR, after tracing their argument's backing, I found that reviewers initially analyzed a total of thirty relevant clinical trials. How did Manser et al. come to exclude more evidence than they included in their review? The reviewers indicate that they excluded evidences from twenty-one trials for one or more of the following reasons.

- The trial did not have a control arm;
- the trial did not report disease-specific mortality for lung cancer as an outcome; and/or
- the trial's duration of follow-up was fewer than five years.

Essentially, twenty-one studies were excluded because they did not meet the methodological rigors set out by the reviewers and the Cochrane Collaboration's procedures as outlined in the *Cochrane Handbook*, the PRISMA checklist, and GRADE criteria.

In a more in-depth examination of Manser et al.'s (2013) excluded trials, I found that the majority did lack a control arm, and two of the excluded studies were characterized as observational studies. Reviewers' resistance to relying on uncontrolled studies exists because such trials do not have a group to which the study's treatment arm can be compared. Yet, my research indicates that as many as one-third of trials in ongoing clinical trials listed in the NIH registry are uncontrolled (Saccà 2010); the majority of these uncontrolled studies are in the area of hematology and oncology (or cancer trials). In fact, many clinical trial researchers extol uncontrolled studies because they are a low-stakes way of investigating a new or interesting clinical observation: "Uncontrolled clinical trials are careful, prospective records of the effect of a treatment in a number of patients. They have a predefined protocol, and measure the changes with carefully chosen tools" (White and Ernst 2001, 112). Moreover, uncontrolled clinical trials are of major significance for studies that measure the efficacy of interventions in alternative medicine (see Derkatch 2016).

Controversy about the merit of uncontrolled trials has a deeply rooted past. Three of the major figures who, as described earlier, ushered in standards characterized by evidence-based medicine and CSRs wrote a letter to the editor of the *New England Journal of Medicine* in 1980 declaring that two recent uncontrolled trials published in the journal were based on nothing more than "anecdotal experience" (Sacks, Kupfer, and Chalmers 1980). They then refer to the methodologies of these studies as defective (1980). In a reply, Hollenberg et al. (1980) argued that uncontrolled studies grant researchers the opportunity to conduct preliminary, cost-effective investigations of the feasibility of a particular intervention. Specifically, "without the encouragement provided by such preliminary evidence, the resources required for a large, controlled clinical trial simply cannot be mobilized" (Hollenberg et al. 1980).

I describe this decades-old debate not to stake a claim on one side or the other about the value or rigor of uncontrolled clinical trials but to demonstrate that the criteria for sifting evidence are far from neutral. Evidential criteria are value-laden declarations of what should or shouldn't count. Seemingly benign in nature, Cochrane checklists exert suasive force in their genred protocol for evidential cut making. Cochrane systematic reviews' parenthetical references to charter documents for authoritative support and handy, to-do list–like checkboxes make invisible the historical, political, and ideological assumptions that undergird criteria for assessing and synthesizing evidence.

### Toulminian Analysis of Prostate Cancer–Screening CSR

Tactics for cancer screening have serious implications for the health and well-being of bodies in flux. Some readers might be aware of the controversy surrounding prostate cancer screening—in particular, claims about the efficacy of the prostate-specific antigen (PSA) test. *Forbes Magazine* published an article titled "PSA Testing Does More Harm Than Good" in which Salzberg (2014) argues that PSA tests yield overdiagnosis of prostate cancer. The author concludes that, "once a man is told he has cancer, there is a strong tendency to treat it, and treatment has serious, often harmful side effects: 20–30 percent of men treated with surgery and radiation will have long-term incontinence and erectile dysfunction" (n.p.). Motivated by similar concerns regarding the overdiagnosis of prostate cancer due to using PSA testing in cancer screening, Ilic et al. (2013) proposed and executed their own CSR to synthesize available evidence about prostate cancer screening. Results from a Toulminian analysis of Ilic et al.'s CSR, "Screening for Prostate Cancer," can be found in table 4.4. Reviewers set out to answer the following question: How effective is prostate cancer screening for men in reducing both prostate cancer–specific and all-cause-related mortality?

Ilic et al.'s (2013) main claim does not include an explicit argument for or against prostate cancer screening. Rather, they argue that, "prior to obtaining a PSA test, men should be informed about the known harms that are frequent, both in the immediate- and long-term, versus the potential for

**Table 4.4 Toulminian Analysis of "Screening for Prostate Cancer"
(Ilic et al. 2013)**

| Toulmin's Construct | Associated Argumentative Move |
|---|---|
| Claim | "Prior to obtaining a PSA test, men should be informed about the known harms that are frequent, both in the immediate- and long-term, versus the potential for a benefit that may occur many years in the future." |
| Grounds | Pooled statistical, meta-analysis of five studies ($n$ = 341,342) indicate that screening does not significantly decrease prostate cancer–specific mortality and is associated with a high degree of overdiagnosis, treatment, and screening-related harms. |
| Warrants | Cochrane review methods (including GRADE, PRISMA, *Cochrane Handbook*). |
| Backing | Original studies. |
| Qualifier | "More research is needed." |
| Rebuttal | Not enough data about black men—in the United States, black men have twice the incidence and risk of dying from prostate cancer. And only 4% of men in trials were nonwhite. Also uncertain about how applicable this claim is for men who have a family history of prostate cancer. |

a benefit that may occur many years in the future" (24). Reviewers ground their claim in statistical analyses of pooled data from original studies; such studies measured the effect that routine prostate cancer screening had on men's mortality rates. Ilic et al. relied on the *Cochrane Handbook* to conduct their review. They drew on only five original studies. From these five studies, 341,342 patients were included. Akin to reviewers in the lung cancer CSR discussed above, Ilic et al. acknowledge the need for additional research. Of interest is Ilic et al.'s acknowledgment of one potential counterargument to their claim after noting that the original studies included in their synthesis represent only a fraction of the affected population: reviewers were hard-pressed to find enough data about black men's experiences with prostate cancer screening. Reviewers' difficulty in finding these data is significant since, in the United States alone, black men have twice the incidence and risk of dying from prostate cancer. Ilic et al. also wonder about how their synthesis might have led to different results if they had access to more clinical trials that included men with a family history of prostate cancer. It is possible that at least some of the two hundred original studies that Ilic et al. excluded from their synthesis might have helped to address concerns expressed in their rebuttal.

On what grounds did Ilic et al. (2013) make evidential exclusions, then? According to reasoning presented in both the body of the review and the review's appendix, reviewers excluded these studies because they did not meet the methodological rigors set forth by the Cochrane Collaboration, per the *Cochrane Handbook*, PRISMA checklist, and GRADE criteria. I investigated further the clinical trials that were excluded, and discovered that the majority of the two hundred excluded trials were characterized as cohort studies, narrative reviews, and descriptive studies. The Cochrane Collaboration calls into question the methodological rigor of these three types of analyses.

*Cohort studies* are studies that, for a certain period of time, follow an otherwise healthy population to see who develops a particular disease. *Narrative reviews* are akin to CSRs except that they are not expected to provide as much detail about how individual trials were assessed methodologically. To conduct a *descriptive study*, researchers collect information without manipulating the environment. Synonymous with descriptive studies are correlational or observational studies. The Office of Human Research Protections defines descriptive studies as any study that is not experimental. While descriptive and cohort studies cannot allow for comparisons between treatment and control arms, they do make it possible to map relationally other important factors for promoting and deterring health (e.g., the relationship between a cancer diagnosis and a patient's geographical location). Additionally, descriptive and cohort studies help determine which variables might be manipulated so as to see an intervention's effect; they are quite generative for researchers who are in the early stages of preparing experimental studies. Here again (as is their job), we see the effects of implicit and explicit value judgments that condition reviewers' evidential cuts—cuts that are based on a study's methodological frame.

Cochrane systematic reviewers' cut-making criteria enact normative stances toward bodies and being. In a way, warrants for CSRs' claims (i.e., the Cochrane Collaboration's methodological values) might be thought of as reviewers' authoritative conscience—an argumentative Jiminy Cricket, if you will—that enforces ideological assumptions about the reliability and usefulness of data. In the case of the prostate cancer CSR, warrants enforced ideological assumptions about the reliability and usefulness of ("mere") observations of relationships between people and the world around them. What might have been learned about such relationships, however? What might Ilic et al. (2013) have gleaned about the effectiveness of prostate cancer–screening techniques by accounting for the relationship between an at-risk body and, for example, living near a contaminated water source? What kinds of valuable conclusions are silenced when reviewers make evidential cuts to data from cohort, narrative, and descriptive studies? Does the knowledge gained from making such evidential cuts outweigh what is lost? Is there even a professional platform on which questions like these might be asked and answered?

## Toulminian Analysis of Breast Cancer–Screening CSR

Arguments about whether women should receive routine mammograms as a way to detect and thereby intervene in breast cancer in its earliest stages is fraught with complexity. As I write this, many news sources have received criticism for reporting various iterations of evidence-based claims against the use of mammography for breast cancer screening. Opponents of mammography for the early detection of breast cancer argue that such a tactic is not only ineffective but also dangerous and financially wasteful. Here again, opponents of such a screening protocol worry about overdiagnosis and subsequent psychological and physical harm. Accordingly, in their CSR, Gøtzsche and Jørgensen (2013) set out to answer the following question: What is the efficacy of screening for breast cancer in reducing breast cancer mortality? Results from a Toulminian analysis of this CSR can be found in table 4.5.

In this particular CSR, reviewers appear reluctant to make a definitive recommendation about whether screening for breast cancer with mammography poses more harm than good. Their overarching claims are twofold. First, Gøtzsche and Jørgensen (2013) argue, "The time has come to re-assess whether universal mammography screening should be recommended for any age group" (17). Second, they make the case that "breast cancer mortality is an unreliable outcome measure in screening trials (and therefore also in cohort studies of the effectiveness of national programmes) and exaggerates the benefit" (17). Gøtzsche and Jørgensen's uncertainty about how to measure or detect "benefit" might sound familiar to readers, since such a conundrum was at the heart of the FDA hearing described at the outset of chapter 3.

Unable to resolve such a conundrum, Gøtzsche and Jørgensen resist making an explicit claim about mammography's efficacy. Rather, they mobilize the clinical trial data from original studies as a way to leverage methodological critiques of such studies. Of all of the CSRs I analyzed in preparation for this chapter and in addition to the CSRs I analyzed previously as part of a

**Table 4.5 Toulminian Analysis of "Screening for Breast Cancer with Mammography" (Gøtzsche and Jørgensen 2013)**

| Toulmin's Construct | Associated Argumentative Move |
|---|---|
| Claims | (1) "We believe that the time has come to re-assess whether universal mammography screening should be recommended for any age group." |
| | (2) "Breast cancer mortality is an unreliable outcome measure in screening trials (and therefore also in cohort studies of the effectiveness of national programmes) and exaggerates the benefit." |
| Grounds | Statistical analysis of nine trials ($n$ = 600,000) indicates that screening reduces breast cancer mortality by 15% but leads to overdiagnosis and overtreatment. |
| Warrants | Cochrane review methods themselves (including GRADE, PRISMA, *Cochrane Handbook*). |
| Backing | Original studies. |
| Qualifier | "More research is needed." |
| Rebuttal | In trials where randomization was suboptimal, there was a significant reduction in breast cancer mortality. |

pilot project, this is the only one that posited methodological implications in the main results of the abstract. This is also the only CSR I analyzed wherein reviewers direct readers to an external, "evidence-based document"—the mammography screening leaflet (Gøtzsche et al. 2009)—that claims to fully inform women about benefits and harms of breast cancer screening. Specifically, Gøtzsche and Jørgensen's (2013) critiques of the methodological rigor of the original studies are grounded in statistical analyses of nine trials, which included 600,000 participants in total. Reviewers' statistical analyses also lead them to conclude that screening does, in fact, reduce breast cancer mortality by 15 percent, but that screening also leads to "overdiagnosis and overtreatment" (2). As was the case with the other two CSRs discussed in this chapter, Gøtzsche and Jørgensen relied on Cochrane review methods (specifically GRADE, PRISMA, and the *Cochrane Handbook*) to warrant claims and offer the standard qualifier that more research is needed (17).

Once more, the authors provide an interesting bit of information in the CSR's Toulminian rebuttal. That is, Gøtzsche and Jørgensen (2013) note as an anticipated counterargument that in trials wherein randomization was considered by Cochrane standards to be suboptimal, rates of breast cancer mortality were, in fact, significantly lower. In other words, when Gøtzsche and Jørgensen loosened the methodologically based cut-making criteria in which the Cochrane Collaboration is so entrenched, results of their syntheses suggested that women who are screened using mammography do, in fact, have lower rates of breast cancer mortality. This is perhaps the most obvious example of how systematic reviewers are hamstrung by cut-making criteria when they are expected to make straightforward final claims about whether certain cancer-screening tactics are effective and safe.

In each of the above examples, systematic reviewers' final claims hinge primarily on Toulminian backing, or methodological rigor and procedurality. Such a finding supports the fundamental hypothesis of this book: backstage, material methods for making evidence matter and mean condition, power, and predict diagnoses and prognoses. Even as systematic reviewers work primarily with discursive and statistical evidences, they cannot escape the effect that the biomedical backstage has on their final claims. It may be time, therefore, to reexamine the Toulminian warrants for systematic reviewers' final claims. Some medical experts—in particular, those who have taken on and sought to discredit opponents of using mammography to screen for breast cancer—have done just that. Critics of the Cochrane Collaboration's fixation on methodological rigor as an argumentative warrant are uncomfortable with how current methods for collecting and analyzing clinical trial data might actually be producing "results that are far less rich than they should be" (Condit 1996, 100). One such critic, Elaine Schattner, a medical doctor and journalist, recently commented on the breast cancer–screening controversy: "A lack of evidence doesn't mean something is untrue. It could be that we (in this case medical scientists, epidemiologists, radiologists, statisticians) have failed to measure the right endpoints, or simply failed to measure what's right about early detection of invasive breast cancer" (2015, n.p.). Here, Schattner asks readers to remain mindful of how clinical trial methodologies might fail to capture the complexity of disease, thereby making all subsequent analyses and syntheses deficient. Argumentative common ground on both sides of the breast cancer–screening debate includes methodological and procedural concerns. For Schattner, endpoints and forms of measurement are at issue. For Gøtzsche and Jørgensen (2013), decisions about patient eligibility and whether samples were randomized adequately are at issue. As was the case in both previous CSR analyses, reviewers leverage their final claims by critiquing the methodological rigor of the original studies. In other words, systematic reviewers' evidential cuts hinge on how authors of that which they're reviewing made evidential cuts.

*

Evidential syntheses are a challenging genre. Systematic reviewers must at once aggregate, assess, and generalize. And they must accomplish this without revealing insensitivity to local, lived conditions of the very people (not the data) included in the original clinical trials. Such insensitivity is hard to avoid since the Cochrane Collaboration defines what *is* based on statistical whitewashing and weighted kappas for measuring inter-author reliability. Fixed-effects models, risk ratios, and sensitivity analyses further flatten original clinical trial data. For all the ways that scholars in material feminisms have sought to make the corporeal body matter so as to "better apprehend how the body in its very materiality plays an *active* role" (Barad 2003, 809), the above procedural cuts work at flattening, devaluing, overlooking, and ignoring "what these bodies are such that inscription is possible" (Grosz 2004, 2).

Prior to systematic reviewers' synthesizing labor, the Cochrane Collaboration had to devise statistical and checklist-like techniques for turning heterogeneous data homogenous and for siphoning off human difference in general. Mol and Mesman (1996) note: "Normative questions don't start *after* the facts, with what *ought* to be done or believed. Instead they start right at the beginning, with the business of framing what *is* the case" (420). For Mol and Mesman, there is a backstage to every backstage. What is the material-discursive, deliberative labor that conditions or frames that which comes to matter—even before systematic reviewers set out to synthesize clinical trial data for cancer screening? How does one even gain access to the layers and layers of backstage shadow work involved in making evidential cuts?

Thus far, I have used Toulmin's model for argumentation to analyze the rhetorical labor that precedes final, evidential syntheses. Toulmin's model makes visible how systematic reviewers build arguments. That is, Toulmin's model helps us understand how, exactly, reviewers set out to invent and argumentatively organize a case for or against a particular cancer-screening recommendation. But Toulmin's body of work doesn't only include strategies for mapping the anatomy of arguments. Toulmin, Rieke, and Janik (1984) attend to the very acts of reasoning involved in the backstage labor when crafting those arguments. In particular, they define reasoning as less "a way of *hitting on new ideas*" than a "way of *testing and sifting ideas critically*" (10; italics in the original).

Each of the above Toulminian analyses indicate that final claims are fortified by complex statistical assessments of a large body of clinical trial data and that evidential cut-making procedures are standardized and streamlined through statistical analyses, review software, and Cochrane-approved heuristics and checklists. What Toulmin's model of argumentation alone does not account for is how reviewers *sift* evidences. In other words, Toulmin's model tells us more about how reviewers "hit on new ideas," but much less about how they "test and sift ideas critically" (Toulmin et al. 1984, 10). How, then, do reviewers embark on the difficult rhetorical labor associated with sifting evidences, making evidential cuts, and finding ways that data can be homogenized for the purpose of evidential comparison? Toulmin et al. argue that there are "critical procedures through which ideas are examined in competition with each other and judged by relevant criteria so as to make it possible for us to arrive at reasonable choices" (17). In each of the above CSRs, more studies were excluded from syntheses than were included. Understanding how evidential cuts were made requires attention to synthesizers' practices of testing and sifting ideas critically.

To summarize, Toulmin's model grants me a cursory understanding of the anatomy of CSRs as an argument and how the *Cochrane Handbook*, PRISMA checklist, and GRADE criteria not only warrant final claims but also act as argumentative heuristics for reviewers. On its own, Toulmin's model does not fully account for the backstage, behind-the-scenes, value-ridden rhetorical reasoning involved in establishing the critical criteria by which evidences are finally tested and sifted. Ultimately, this act of deciding on and deploying specific criteria to reason about, sift, and test competing evidences lies at the heart of evidential synthesis as a method for negotiating medical indeterminacy. Thus far, it is unclear how, exactly, reviewers ensure that their statistically sound evidential cuts (as warrants) will be rich enough to withstand the weight of a final claim—a claim that could change the outcome of a patient's health and well-being.

### Supplementing Toulminian Analyses with Stasis Theory

I hypothesize that stasis theory can provide us with a language for capturing the complexity of the backstage, ideological, cut-making labor involved in evidential syntheses. In the second century B.C., Hermagoras introduced stases as a way of categorizing moments in an argument when contention or points of disagreement revealed themselves. Later, in *De Inventione*, *Institutio Oratoria*, and *On Stases*, Cicero, Quintillian, and Hermogenes (see Nadeau 1964), respectively, more explicitly proposed the rhetorical value of using stases as heuristics.[6] That is, stases can be used to taxonomize arguments into one or more of four basic questions:

- questions of fact (or conjecture)
- questions of definition
- questions of value (or quality)
- questions of procedure (or translation, jurisdiction)

Fahnestock and Secor (1988) argue that stases can be seen "as sitting between the general outline of an argument, applicable to all arguments regardless of field, described by the Toulmin model, and the very specific lines of argument engendered by the special topoi preferred by specific disciplines" (429). Stases can point to that which motivates or conditions a particular investigation. Stases can also point to when an investigation or debate reaches a kind of argumentative standstill. As Walsh and Walker (2013) remind readers, "stasis" in Latin means sticking points, steps, or levels. Prelli's (1989) modifications to stasis theory equip researchers interested in analyzing scientific sticking points. Building on Prelli's version of stasis theory, Northcut (2007) modifies classical and contemporary versions of stasis theory in order to understand how scientific indeterminacies are ultimately resolved. She acknowledges that, in the sciences, "claims tend to be hypotheses, and arguments are rarely resolved with absolute certainty" (1) and that "stasis works best when modified to fit the discourse norms of specialized fields" (3). While for Prelli and Northcut stases indicate moments of stoppage or an argumentative point wherein "conflict must be resolved in order for further discussion to be relevant" (Northcut 2007, 4), when paired with Toulmin's argumentative parts of speech, I propose that stasis theory can help identify moments of evidential cut making.

Pairing Toulmin's model for argumentation with a modified version of stasis theory captures the rhetorical complexity of reviewers' backstage, synthesizing labor—or what Happe (2013) might refer to as the "political unconscious" that "underlies the theories and methods of science" (10). Stasis theory helps us unearth practices of sifting and reasoning that make up the rhetorical bedrock of systematic reviewers' argumentative backstage. Figure 4.6 is an analytic heuristic for analyzing the rhetorical labor characteristic of evidential synthesis. Whereas the final claim, or "destination," of the CSR is a recommendation (*not* a certitude) about the efficacy of a particular cancer-screening technique, and the rest of the review consists of Toulminian grounds, or answers to the anticipated question, "What've you got to go on?" we see that the overwhelming majority of CSRs rest at the stasis of procedure.

While the grounds of CSRs rest at the stasis of procedure, their backing (or methods used in the original studies) may rest at any one or more of

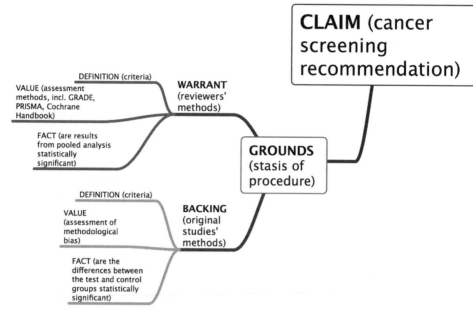

Figure 4.6 Toulminian-stasis analytic heuristic (modified for analyzing CSRs)

the following stases: definition (or cut-making criteria deployed by original studies); value (an assessment of original studies' methodological biases); and fact (an assertion that individual, original studies' results either are or are not statistically significant). Final recommendations about cancer screening's efficacy are warranted by actual CSR reviewers' methods themselves. They, too, might involve periodic halts in the argumentation through definition (reviewers' criteria for inclusion/exclusion); value (reviewers own assessment methods, including GRADE, PRISMA, and the *Cochrane Handbook*); and/or fact (reviewers' assertion that results from pooled analysis are or are not statistically significant).

Evidential syntheses require systematic reviewers to collate large swaths of independent evidence from studies that were conducted very differently (i.e., researchers collected and assessed results differently). The authors of CSRs, therefore, must find ways to turn each of these very different data points into a stabilized (for now) collection of comparable evidences. This is, after all, what it means to "synthesize." In each study that systematic reviewers consider for possible inclusion, they contend with variations in

- investigative apparatuses;
- research questions;

- assessment methods;
- the health of individual participants; and
- individual participants' demographics.

Resolving these variations means resolving a series of scientific sticking points. Based on analyses of the above three cancer-screening CSRs, reviewers make evidential cuts in the face of biological and procedural indeterminacy at the following sticking points.

- Stases of *fact* require that reviewers negotiate answers to questions about whether findings (from either original studies or their synthesis) are statistically significant.
- Stases of *definition* require that reviewers negotiate answers to questions about preanalysis criteria devised to standardize which original studies, collection techniques, and participants will be included (in the original studies or their synthesis).
- Stases of *value* require that reviewers negotiate answers to questions about methodological rigor (of the original studies or their synthesis).

What I'm arguing here is that it is not enough to assert (and subsequently critique, if one is so inclined) that systematic reviewers are forced into limiting their claims about the efficacy of a particular cancer-screening approach based on methodological grounds. As illustrated in figure 4.6, limits to claims about a particular screening intervention are rooted even more deeply in reviewers' evidential cuts regarding statistical significance of original studies, biases of original studies, statistical significance of pooled analyses, and the authoritativeness of assessment apparatuses such as GRADE and the *Cochrane Handbook*.

Unearthing each of the above stases helps us to account for and name what fortifies (and fails to fortify) systematic reviewers' final claims. For example, my analyses indicate that none of the CSRs made evidential cuts based on how (and by whom) original studies were funded. And none of the CSRs I analyzed made evidential cuts based on the demographic, socioeconomic, or geographic generalizability of the findings of individual studies. In other words, when examining evidential syntheses, it is as important to notice and name that which is not included as it is to identify that which is. Evidential cuts help resolve questions about how (and how well) *we* did what we did and how (and how well) *they* did what they did. Understanding the complexity of these cuts requires attending not just to their argumentative anatomy but also to how warrants and backing, by fetishizing only certain questions related to definition, value, and fact, obscure the ideological and political assumptions implicit in cut-making criteria. Stasis theory helps us access the assumptions and values left unaccounted for by Toulmin's model.

## CUT-MAKING CRITIQUES

For those holding their breath while living in a constant state of prognosis (Jain 2007)—those who remain ever vigilant by "seeking out lurking disease before it can ambush us" (Belling 2010, 231)—proper cancer-screening protocols are intended to provide a kind of authoritative exhale. When determining best cancer-screening practices, making evidential cuts helps resolve indeterminacies, but only those indeterminacies that are deemed most meaningful. Paradoxically, the claims that CSR reviewers make rely on assessing and making transparent procedural infrastructures, and yet the very value-laden, cut-making criteria that inform such infrastructural critiques are so weaved "into the fabric of everyday life" (Weiser 1991, 94) that they, themselves, have become invisible. As the epigraph to this chapter indicates, we ought to ask more frequently about "constraints that infrastructures impose, and the forms of erasure and homogenization in which they engage" (Dourish and Bell 2011, 95).

In the opening pages of this book, I asked: Whose evidence counts, and how? This chapter provides readers with some idea of how decisions about evidential cuts hinge on disciplinary and methodological standards. This chapter also demonstrates how "standards are both technical *and* moral projects" (Busch 2011, 286). It's plausible that some readers did not need the analyses above to understand CSRs as what some in the medical community refer to as methodological fetishism (Greenhalgh and Russell 2006). What my analyses do demonstrate, however, is the rhetorical nature of emerging standards of care. Busch (2011) has made the case that standards are "almost invariably the result of conflict or disagreement" (33). And indeed, in the case of CSRs, there is a good deal of scientifically resolved disagreement buried in their appendices and sedimented in the Cochrane Collaboration's handbook, PRISMA statement, and GRADE criteria. The exact degree to which some data are silenced through flat out erasure or homogenization is yet to be determined. The effect of these erasures and homogenizations on actual lived experiences of real people is also yet to be determined.

The desire to practice medicine in a way that values methodological rigor is not in and of itself particularly egregious. The billions of dollars spent per year in the United States alone on medical malpractice liability (e.g., insurance, awards, and administrative costs not covered by insurance) points to both an implicit and explicit demand for expert, accurate, and evidence-based medical practice. What, then, is the relationship between care and managed accountability? Greenhalgh and Russell (2006) pose a similar, albeit slightly more provocative question: "Is the methodological fetishism of which the Cochrane Collaboration has been accused an extreme example of the politicization of science by the new managerialists?" (37).

Using rhetorical theory to unpack the argumentative power of methodological matters gives us an opportunity to reimagine how other, nonstandardized evidences could be made to mean in medical practice. Derkatch (2008) makes the case that method—specifically, the randomized, well-controlled clinical trial—acts as a boundary object that maintains biomedicine's authoritative ethos amid competing ways of practicing care (e.g., alternative medicine). Derkatch (2008) invokes Michael Gorman's notion of an "élite" trading zone "where a group of experts use their specialized knowledge to dictate how a socio-technical system will function" (384). Gorman (2002) indicates that such specialized expertise is "black-boxed for other participants in the network" (933). I hope that this chapter has helped prop open one such black box in medical practice. Additionally, I hope that this chapter has laid the theoretical groundwork for methodological revisions to evidential syntheses—revisions that may make it possible to attune to many and varied sources of evidence.

The risk of failing to attune to heterogeneous sources and assessments of evidence when synthesizing final claims is not just that some voices will not be heard or that some bodies will not be counted. The risk of failing to attune to multiple material sources and assessments of evidence when synthesizing final claims is not just an affront to narratives that champion individual choice and patient empowerment. The risk of syntheses that attune rhetorically only to some evidence and not others is that in an effort to "find out what we know already" (Chalmers et al. 2014), we fail to understand what it is we *do not yet know*. One critic of CSRs refers to such a phenomenon as a conceptual cul-de-sac. Specifically, Greenhalgh argues, "researchers in dominant paradigms tend to be very keen on procedure. They set up committees to define and police the rules of their paradigm, awarding grants and accolades to those who follow those rules. This entire circular exercise works very well just after the establishment of a new paradigm, since building systematically on what has gone before is an efficient and effective route to scientific progress. But once new discoveries have stretched the paradigm to its limits, these same rules and procedures become counterproductive and constraining. That's what I mean by conceptual cul-de-sacs" (2012, 93). Greenhalgh's critique echoes with greater specificity Harding's (2006) argument that science's methods and claims are not, in fact, value free. Reviewers' methodological critiques cloak how handbooks, heuristics, and computational partners exert ideological force and might be guiding medical practitioners round and round conceptual cul-de-sac after conceptual cul-de-sac.

The crisis of the conceptual cul-de-sac transcends discipline. Barthes (1986) bemoans that, even for writers, "method becomes a law" and "nothing remains for the writing" (318). In response, Butler (1994) encourages us to acknowledge that foundations are always contingent. Critics of CSRs like Greenhalgh, Howick, and Maskrey (2014) argue that "tools that contain quantitative estimates of risk and benefit are needed"; however, such tools "must be designed to support conversations not climb probability trees" (n.p.). Petticrew and Egan (2006) use the term "floccinaucinihilipilification" to describe "the process by which a great deal of the evidence available to illuminate an issue is defined as worthless because it does not fit into an evidence hierarchy or cannot be synthesized using available methods" (quoted in Popay 2006, 76). As demonstrated both here and in chapter 3, conversations are, indeed, cut short when only certain kinds of evidences may be invoked as grounds during evidential assessment.

The truest test of how well a method for evidential synthesis is attuned to bodies in flux will be how it manages and accounts for qualitative evidences. Dixon-Woods et al. (2006) wonder "whether the template offered by conventional systematic review methodology can comfortably accommodate qualitative research" (31). Similarly, Lucas et al. (2007) argue, "further methodological work is required on the processes by which evidence from studies using different qualitative methods and generating a range of types of evidence can be synthesized and combined with quantitative findings on effect without compromising the need to minimize bias" (quoted in Higgins and Green [2011], sec. 20.3.2.5). Might there be an opportunity here for collaborations between technical communicators, rhetoricians, and medical scientists who design clinical trials and synthesize evidences? Might the kinds of rhetorical-analytic labor demonstrated in the analyses above be useful to medical professionals who desire to include qualitative evidences in their syntheses? Might technical communicators and rhetoricians — experts at making the strange familiar — contribute nuanced ways of making count that which is currently characterized as uncountable?

Changes in evidence-based medical standards, cancer-screening techniques, and subsequent clinical practice might, indeed, be theorized as a Kuhnian paradigm shift, but the cut-making practices demonstrated above suggest that these changes are also the result of rhetorical negotiations and Fleckian thought collectives. Ideally, Fleckian thought collectives should help account for "pluricentric collectives with different gravity centers and degrees of closure" (Peine 2011, 503). Syntheses of both quantitative and qualitative evidences pose the problem of how to negotiate varying gravity centers and degrees of closure.

Surely, rhetoricians, technical communicators, social scientists, and medical professionals could work together to resolve procedural sticking points, resist conceptual cul-de-sacs, and sanction the validity of pluricentric collectives. After all, in this chapter I have just demonstrated how classical and contemporary rhetorical theory can be paired productively as an analytic lens for understanding evidential cut-making practices. Fahnestock and Secor (1988) have argued that "the usefulness of classical rhetoric is often extolled but less often demonstrated" (427). And yet, rhetorical theory can be used "as an instrument capable of performing ... intricate analysis" (427). Given our strengths in analytic reasoning and writing, scholars in rhetoric and technical communication ought to seek out collaborations with medical scientists and clinicians and to assist in revisions to standardized strategies for assessing methodological procedures—revisions that enact the pluricentric nature of biomedical practice and scientific progress, in general.

# 5. COMPUTING EVIDENCE

*Core to our philosophy is customer choice and empowerment through data.*
Anne Wojcicki, CEO, 23andMe, Inc.

*Genes are "material-semiotic object[s] of knowledge" that are*
*"forged by heterogeneous practices in the furnaces of technoscience."*
Donna Haraway, *Modest_Witness@Second_Millennium.*
*FemaleMan©_Meets_OncoMouse*™

Only 5–10 percent of breast cancers in the United States are linked to an inherited genetic mutation, but in the last year almost one hundred thousand women in the United States alone have requested genetic testing for mutations that are correlated with an increase in breast and ovarian cancer.[1] In addition to the Angelina Jolie effect described in chapter 1, there are several other factors that may encourage otherwise healthy women to seek out genetic testing. First, genetic testing is more accessible than ever before. As of August 1, 2012, the Affordable Care Act requires that insurance plans must cover genetic testing costs. Second, genetic testing is more affordable than ever before. Since 2013, the genetic test for BRCA mutations has decreased from $3,000 to, in some cases, as low as $200. Finally, many evidence-based medical professionals are convinced that the new frontier of genetic evidence poses great predictive power.

Genetic evidence is praised for the ways it makes possible more personalized, "patient-powered" health care. Recently, in fact, President Obama declared a "precision medicine initiative"—a "bold new research effort to revolutionize how we improve health and treat disease" ("Fact Sheet," 2015), based largely on genomic analyses. "Launched with a $215 million investment in the President's 2016 Budget, the Precision Medicine Initiative will pioneer a new model of patient-powered research that promises to accelerate biomedical discoveries and provide clinicians with new tools, knowledge, and therapies to select which treatments will work best for which patients" ("Fact Sheet," 2015). The promise of precision medicine could, indeed, help ameliorate concerns about medical protocols that are based on fictional, "average" patients (see chap. 3 for an in-depth discussion about the limitations of statistically rendered assessments based on population data). For oncologists, precision medicine promises to transform how cancers such as breast and ovarian cancers can be treated: "Patients with breast, lung, and colorectal cancers, as well as melanomas and leukemias, for instance, routinely undergo molecular testing as part of patient care, enabling physicians to select treatments that improve chances of survival and reduce exposure to adverse effects" ("Fact Sheet," 2015). The White House claims that precision medicine "will leverage advances in genomics, emerging methods for managing and analyzing large data sets while protecting privacy, and health information technology to accelerate biomedical discoveries" ("Fact Sheet," 2015). The general public knows little about what lies beneath genetic evidence's political and economic substrates—in particular, the computational methods that genetic scientists use to navigate and make sense of enormous data sets.

While increased affordability and access to genetic testing along with the promise of personalized and more precise medical practice certainly sounds like scientific progress, recent research indicates an alarming statistic: nearly two-thirds of women who request testing for genetic mutations correlated with an increase in breast and ovarian cancer do not receive genetic counseling (Armstrong et al. 2015). This means that while tens of thousands of women are provided information about their bodies that may have serious implications for decisions they make about their health—including the preventative bilateral mastectomies I discussed in chapter 4—a majority of women are choosing to forgo the counseling and medical expertise that would assist and support them in translating findings from genetic tests.

Such statistics are not only alarming to the medical community; they are a call to action for technical communicators and rhetoricians. Those who study and teach rhetorically sound technical communication have long been concerned with ethical and effective methods for translating and rendering risk palpable and probable. When I, myself, investigated the possibility of purchasing an at-home genetic testing kit, I realized how little I knew about the computational methods with which risks are translated and rendered palpable and probable. Motivated by Latour and Woolgar's (1986) assertions regarding "the importance of the material elements of the laboratory in the production of facts" (238) and that "the process of construction involves the use of certain devices whereby all traces of production are made extremely difficult to detect" (176), in this chapter I analyze direct-to-consumer genetic sequencing's computational methods for negotiating medical uncertainty. Mindful of the technical, rhetorical, and public health implications associated with so-called personalized, precision medicine, I map how genetic evidences come into being (Daston 2000).

Up until this point I have bracketed in-depth discussions of the economic conditions associated with the biomedical backstage's material-discursive labor. In this chapter, however, I explore the ideological, economic, and algorithmic machines that make genetic information meaningful. I hope that by unearthing the evidential shadow work involved in computing genetic evidence, readers might feel more prepared to interrogate politicized promises of a more personalized and precise approach to medical practice. I hope, too, that this chapter helps make readers who are considering genetic testing more aware of the complexity associated with computing and commoditizing human DNA—especially readers who plan to circumvent doctors and genetic counselors completely by ordering genetic testing kits online.

I stand, in this chapter, on the shoulders of others who continue to critique the black-boxed labor involved in commoditizing DNA as evidence. Kramer (2015) describes how most genetic genealogical tests, while assumedly truthful, objective, and cutting edge, "are but partial and incomplete, as they only chart male lines of descent through surname or one-name research" (88). Parthasarathy's (2012) book, *Building Genetic Medicine*, highlights how the variety of differing transnational techniques and approaches to breast cancer genetic science have shaped the very practice of genetic science, thereby influencing how we come to know about, name, and predict our genetic futures. Such differences have a profound effect on "how risks and disease are being defined and redefined" (Parthasarathy 2012, 3). Recall that I began this book by referencing the premodern medical practice of astrological contemplation, or stargazing, as a way of making corporeal predictions; Parthasarathy ends her book by reminding us that one of the scientists responsible for the "discovery" of the structure of DNA, James Watson, once said, "We used to think our future was in the stars. Now we know our future is in the genes" (199). In this chapter, I extend Parthasarathy's departure from such an assertion and concur that, indeed, "our genomic futures are by no means preordained"; rather, "the way genetics is understood, genetic technologies developed, and genetic medicine is built is ... fundamentally shaped by national social and political context" (199). Put simply: genetic evidences are mutually constituted or coconstructed materials. To truly understand how genetic evidences gain suasive power and help people "do things with things" (Barnett and Boyle 2016), it helps to unearth their socioeconomic, political bedrock.

In an analysis of how a biopharmaceutical company called Myriad Genetics marketed their BRACAnalysis product to consumers, Majdik and Platt (2012) determined that while shrouded in the promise of empowerment, Myriad marketed to healthy women who were worried about their cancer risk by deploying an irrefutable sense of moral urgency and obligation. Women were encouraged "to empower themselves with the information they need to make informed decisions about medical choices," but Majdik and Platt detailed how that sense of empowerment "comes with a price" (137). And that price is not just financial. The transfer of biomedical evidence from the laboratory into the for-profit private sector carries with it serious affective and ideological consequences, including what Majdik and Platt call a gendered sense of moral urgency.

Other scholars similarly critique the ethical-ideological consequences of genetic testing's socioeconomic and political backstage shadow work. Happe (2013) attends to historical linkages "between genomics and the economic and social order" (23) by reminding readers of genomics' historical, material, and ideological roots: eugenics (see also Condit 1999). After analyzing media reports, scientific studies, regulatory texts, and other dominant discourses that circulate around genetics as scientific progress, Happe characterizes the project from which genetic testing hails—the Human Genome Project (HGP)—as "a product of the social and political culture of the 1980s, all the while bearing traces of eugenicist ideology" (46). Happe highlights the fraught nature of the HGP from its very inception. "The history of the HGP reflects the culmination of many converging institutional interests, interests that prevailed because their opponents' arguments were limited to the technical sphere; because social discourse was virtually nonexistent, thanks to the privileged status of reasoning in the technical sphere; and because the ELSI [Ethical, Legal, and Social Implications] program had been unilaterally established by Watson" (45–46). She builds a case about how narratives of "health and illness" are, as were narratives during the eugenics movement, "dependent on the conceptual transfer of causal power from the economic to the genetic, as well as on a particular gendered, racialized, and privatized social order" (24). Happe's discourse analyses reveal genetic science's "value-laden way of describing bodies, environments, and social relations" (21). This chapter takes Happe's work a step further by examining how such value-laden ways of describing bodies, environments, and social relations are actually built into genetic scientists' backstage, material-discursive labor—labor that conditions and commoditizes corporeal futures.

Well aware of the layers of actors and actants involved in the computation of genetic fact, the Center for Disease Control and Prevention (CDC) warns the public that "genetic tests for many diseases are developed on the basis of limited scientific information and may not yet provide valid or useful results to individuals who are tested" (CDC 2015). The CDC explicitly warns citizens about the risks of direct-to-consumer genetic testing: "Many genetic tests are being marketed prematurely to the public through the Internet, TV, and other media. This may lead to the misuse of these tests and the potential for physical or psychological harms to the public" (CDC 2015). The FDA decided recently that the best way to measure the risk associated with genetic testing is to assess consequences of reporting a false result.[2] The potential for false results is quite high—especially results from direct-to-consumer genetic testing companies who, because of regulatory lag, are not operating under the same standard as other genetic sequencing companies. Despite a plethora of regulatory warnings and politicized rhetorics about genetic testing, consumers like myself are largely unaware of the algorithmic labor and technical expertise associated with backstage methods for genetic sequencing. Since "the value of" genetic tests "are in part guaranteed by the techniques by which results are procured" (Kramer 2015, 82), it makes sense to take time to investigate what, exactly, those techniques are. The invisibility of this labor complicates consumers' capacity to assess how (and whether) these evidences warrant not only financial investment but also health-related actions and interventions.

The tools, technologies, and techniques I go on to interrogate in this chapter have social, political, and material histories (see app. C for a brief summary of genetic sequencing methods and associated techniques that precede what is now referred to as next-generation genetic sequencing). According to Lee et al. (2013), gel electrophoresis, paper/column chromatography, and X-ray diffraction were the three most popular and meaningful discoveries leading up to contemporary genetic testing methods. Many of these techniques are based on agential assumptions similar to those described in chapter 2. That is, scientists in the biomedical backstage leverage the agential capacity of nonhuman and not-quite-human (Bennett 2010) objects (e.g., fluorescent dyes, beads, radioactive markers) whose intra-actions (Barad 2007) yield evidences that are then summed up discursively. But results from genetic sequencing hail not just from behind-the-scenes material intra-actions. Genetic evidences are also the consequence of fraught political and socioeconomic milieus.

Direct-to-consumer genetic testing involves dominant discourses (see also Condit 1999; Pender 2012) and a host of "mundane architectures and economies" (Lynch 2013), each of which uniquely shapes how medical professionals negotiate medical uncertainty. Lynch (2013) builds on scholarship in science and technology studies to argue that "inventorying the furniture of the world and outlining how we may come to know about it no longer is the privilege of philosophical reflection" (3). In this chapter, I extend and amplify Happe's (2013) critiques by pairing them with Lynch's suggestion that we "mundanize epistemology, ontology, ethics and aesthetics" to trace central concepts' "historicized and situated" nature (2–3). Rickert's (2013) construct, ambient rhetoric, assumes that there are "conditions that give rise to our ongoing perceptions and understandings of the world" (xiii) and that "nonhuman aspects of place are both more dynamic and more integrated into our practices than we have recognized them to be" (43). If we can agree that matter, movement, and time have significant consequences on human bodies— what Alaimo (2008) might refer to as "trans-corporeality" (238)—then how we account for matter, movement, and time's effects requires nuanced methodological approaches. Methodological approaches should enable analyses that document "rich, complex modes of analysis that travel through the entangled territories of material and discursive, natural and cultural, biological and textual" (Alaimo 2008, 238). This chapter enacts such analytic methods. In particular, I am mindful of how backstage labor associated with computing evidence from billions of petabits of genetic data begs for constant critical attention since, as Jasanoff (2004) argues, "What happens in science and technology today is interwoven with issues of meaning, values, and power in ways that demand sustained critical inquiry" (29).[3] As I've stated elsewhere, methods matter.

### MACHINATIONS OF GENETIC TESTING

As the CDC, FDA, and other government agencies struggle to keep up with the high rate at which genomic science evolves from day to day, consumers concerned about their genetic risk for developing certain cancers are caught in the crossfire. A senior director of bioinformatics products at Thermo Fisher (whose website states they are the "world leader in serving science") admits that "our ability to measure outweighs our ability to interpret and apply" (Buguliskis 2015). It would seem, therefore, that regulatory lag is not the only problem that complicates how informed consumers are about the risks of genetic testing. Consumers must also be aware of analytical lag. Because genetic testing companies have more information than they know how to handle they have developed nuanced (and proprietary) computational techniques. One such technique—next-generation genetic sequencing—specializes in analyzing extremely large data sets. To manage the sheer magnitude of these data, next-generation genetic sequencing techniques require coproduced algorithms, procedures, and machines. These are contemporary medical rhetorics.

Unveiling the relationship among algorithms, machines, and rhetoric is a necessary first step for understanding computational analyses in genetic science. James J. Brown Jr. (2014) defines rhetoric as "a collection of machines ('whatsits,' 'gadgets') for generating and interpreting arguments" (496). In addition to Erasmus's *copia* and Ian Bogost's (2007) procedural rhetoric, Brown (2014) builds on Rice's (2008) discussion of rhetoric as machinic, Kennedy's (2010) articulation of Wikipedia's bots as agentic, and Brock's

(2012) argument that "semantic and computational codes" afford "generative and mutating creations of meaning and interpretation" (n.p.). Computational rhetorics, therefore, are algorithms and procedures for making sense. They act as a "difference engine" that "exerts force on the world" (Brown 2014, 505, 506). Brown claims that "all rhetorical action … is machinic" (498) and proposes the productive possibility of "robot rhetors" (e.g., "software that composes news stories and academic articles, Google search algorithms" [511]). Rather than reducing rhetorical action as machinic and rhetors as robots to a form of Heideggerian enframement, however, Brown notes how computational rhetoric's coproductive nature (i.e., "these machines are simultaneously authoring and authored, writing and written" [p. 509]) presents possibilities for local, contextual, and emergent sense making. Brown's notion of computational rhetorics is particularly useful for my purposes in this chapter in that it lends theoretical support for unpacking how the indeterminacy of human health posed by bodies in flux is managed through computational analyses of large data sets.

Two direct-to-consumer genetic testing companies in particular—23andMe, Inc., and Color Genomics, Inc.—are my objects of analyses in this chapter. Web presences and advertising campaigns for both 23andMe and Color Genomics are impressive, stylish, and suasive. Both companies appeal to consumers by boasting that their products allow for individual empowerment and medical choice making. On their website, 23andMe states: "We bring your genetics to you." That is, consumers can perform the collection of genetic data in the comfort of their own home, ship samples of their genetic data off to a laboratory in prepaid packaging, and several weeks later receive results—all without the hassle of an intermediary human being.

One would assume that both 23andMe's and Color Genomics's laboratories employ similar techniques when analyzing the genetic data that consumers send in for analysis. I was surprised to learn, however, that this is not the case. Even though both corporations highlight in their advertisements that they offer genetic testing for a wide variety of factors, their actual methods for conducting those tests are quite different. These procedural differences have important implications for how we understand contemporary biomedical practices and computational rhetorics. Before I detail such differences, below I provide readers with relevant background information about 23andMe and Color Genomics.

### 23andMe

Among the dozens of direct-to-consumer genetic testing companies, readers are likely familiar with 23andMe because of recent media attention and regulatory scrutiny. In 2013, the FDA ordered 23andMe to cease marketing their personal genome service product in the United States. In a rather stern warning letter (dated November 22, 2013), the FDA indicated that 23andMe was "marketing the 23andMe Saliva Collection Kit and Personal Genome Service (PGS) without marketing clearance or approval in violation of the Federal Food, Drug and Cosmetic Act" (U.S. FDA 2013). Additionally, the FDA argued that uses for the personal genome service that 23andMe listed on their website fall under the definition of a medical device, per 201(h) of the U.S. Federal Food, Drug, and Cosmetic Act—but uses articulated in 201(h) had not yet been officially classified.[4] Subsequently, 23andMe needed to obtain "premarket approval or de novo classification." Because 23andMe failed to comply with requirements associated with obtaining regulatory approval for this innovative technology, and due to the potential danger associated with consumers receiving false positives or negatives about their genetic risk for particularly alarming conditions (e.g., BRCA-related genetic risks and drug responses), the FDA ordered that 23andMe "immediately discontinue marketing the PGS until such time as it receives FDA marketing authorization for the device." However, in a shocking turn of events, 23andMe was recently permitted to market in the United States their personal genome service for detecting genetic markers characteristic of Bloom syndrome, an inherited disorder associated with (among other embodied effects) a significantly increased risk of cancer. And as of January 2016, 23andMe is now compliant with the FDA's rules on how to classify and market at-home genetic testing kits for $199. Consumers' test results state clearly: "Our tests do not diagnose any health conditions."[5] It is my understanding that as of January 2016, 23andMe can no longer report results from BRCA analysis or report the likelihood that a consumer would develop Alzheimer's disease.

The hallmark (and what some see as the main benefit) of direct-to-consumer genetic testing kits like those from 23andMe is that a physician's supervision or approval is not required. This is one of the reasons why narratives of individual empowerment circulate so readily around direct-to-consumer genetic testing kits. Such narratives are persuasive even to me. After years of suffering from seemingly invisible (to others) symptoms associated with thyroid disorders and migraine headaches, I often resist seeking medical attention for fear that my primary care physician will label me hypochondriacal (for more on this, see Segal's [2005] chapter titled "Hypochondria as a Rhetorical Disorder"). Direct-to-consumer genetic testing relieves me of the anxiety that emerges when I think about having to justify to an expert my pervasive concern about a deadly inherited genetic legacy. Moreover, I don't have to agonize about whether my insurance company will pay for the test. This product truly is, as some direct-to-consumer genetic testing corporations have marketed it, a concierge service. While it is easy to be lured in by the promise of "the comfort of my own home," it's important to remember that much if not all of actual DNA analyses happen in a laboratory many miles away from home. And the reference populations to which genetic scientists will compare my genetic data are sourced many more miles away. Readers will come to understand how significant time, space, and movement are for the computation of genetic evidence in the biomedical backstage.

## Color Genomics

Color Genomics provides a genetic testing kit for $249 that, although it does require a physician's order, is mailed directly to the consumer's home. This start-up direct-to-consumer genetic testing company has successfully married computer science expertise with biology expertise. In a sea of direct-to-consumer genetic testing kits, Othman Laraki, a cofounder of Color Genomics, wisely differentiates his product from its competitors with a statement on the company's blog that their "mission is to democratize access to genetic testing."[6] And, indeed, Color Genomics has found ways to make the test free to lower-income communities. What's unique about Color Genomics's product is that they boast expertise in detecting genetic risks for breast and ovarian cancers.[7] On Color Genomics's website are persuasive personal statements from young women, such as: "Taking a proactive stance on my health is totally empowering. It makes me the informed decision maker." Color Genomics also includes on their website a quote from Angelina Jolie's *New York Times* op-ed: "It has got to be a priority to ensure that more women can access gene testing and lifesaving preventive treatment, whatever their means and background, wherever they live" (Jolie 2013). Color Genomics highlights access and affordability as crucial to care.

Evidence that Color Genomics provides to consumers is similar to evidences on which Angelina Jolie based her decision to have a preventative double mastectomy and, more recently, a laparoscopic bilateral salpingo-oophorectomy (removal of ovaries and fallopian tubes). According to several studies, these kinds of preventative surgeries are on the rise, despite findings that such surgeries don't actually improve survival rates (e.g., Tuttle et al. 2007; Jones et al. 2009). Dahl (2016) notes that

> this type of finding is usually reported, by medical experts and veteran health journalists alike, with a finger-wagging tone. Don't these women *know* they're taking an unnecessary risk by choosing a surgery with potential harms that don't outweigh the benefits? But this attitude

at least partially misses the point, by overlooking the role psychology plays in making this hugely difficult medical choice. Uncertainty, for example, is a terrifically difficult state of mind to live with. One classic study in the 1960s suggested that if you give people the option of definitely receiving a painful electric shock right now, or *maybe*—but maybe not—receiving one several moments from now, most will choose the former option. The devil you know, et cetera.

Dahl's assertion that "uncertainty . . . is a terrifically difficult state of mind to live with" lies at the heart of direct-to-consumer genetic testing's success. And yet, I wonder how many who look to genetic evidence to mitigate such uncertainty understand the unwieldy and contingent nature of genetic evidences themselves.

### METHODOLOGICAL RATIONALE

Medical rhetoricians frequently analyze written genres and discourses when making claims about how evidences are leveraged during decision and public policy making (cf. Happe 2013; Mebust and Katz 2008; Popham and Graham 2008; Schryer, Lingard, and Spafford 2005; Teston 2009). Analytic attention is less often paid to predeliberative, material-discursive designs of medical evidences as writing or rhetoric. Limiting our analytic gaze to final discursive representations of medical practices "produces results that are far less rich than they should be" (Condit 1996, 100). Even Happe's (2013) rhetorical method, while rooted in a rich cultural studies tradition, assumes that "discourse is the means by which dominant ideas are both circulated as common sense and shared among otherwise contrary interests" (17); she does not consider the role of the technological missing masses (Latour 1992) that are frequently elided as merely epiphenomenal to scientific knowledge.[8] One way to extend work like Happe's and thereby prop open the black box of how evidences are computed in direct-to-consumer genetic sequencing is to analyze specific companies' backstage technical and analytic labor—labor that is both discursive *and* material, human *and* not-quite-human (Bennett 2010, ix).

Earlier scholars' attempts at understanding how genetic evidence is constructed have involved a wide range of objects of study. Several scholars frame the gene itself as an object of study, including Haraway who, drawing on Marxist theories of materiality, describes the gene as a fetishized commodity. TallBear (2013) similarly describes genes as commodities that are "seen as autonomous, objective things," thereby "obscuring and displacing the social relations between the humans and . . . nonhumans involved in the production of such objects" (70). I take to be true Spinuzzi's (2011; citing Engeström

2006) argument that objects are "embedded in multiple activities simultaneously" and "have lives of their own that resist goal-rational attempts at control and prediction" (194). Connolly (2013) similarly describes how objects have their own systems of self-organization. Given the messy and complex coproduction of genetic evidences and that "the human is always intermeshed with the more-than-human world" (Alaimo 2008, 238), one methodological solution to the problem of studying the genomic backstage is to deploy a version of grounded theory that does not isolate an object of study, such as the gene, from its environment. Rather, I embrace a tactic that allows me to more holistically account for heretofore uninterrogated and overlapping contributors to genetic evidences, including bodies, biologies, geographies, and technologies.

Next-generation genetic sequencing is a complicated computational method for corralling genetic objects and medical indeterminacy. An early methodological attempt at mapping as many contributors as possible to the work of direct-to-consumer genetic testing can be found in figure 5.1. This map soon became unwieldy. I needed a more disciplined method for capturing the fluid and dynamic relationships and intersections between bodies, biologies, geographies, and technologies. Because both Haraway (2008) and Jasanoff (2004) describe genetic evidences as coconstituted objects (cf. Latour 1993), I needed to account for how (a) genetic science and society coproduce or intersect with one another, and (b) genetic scientists and those on whom they rely for samples of genetic information coproduce or intersect with genetic evidences. Toward those ends, this chapter deploys a version of Clarke's (2005) situational analysis—a modification to grounded theory "after the postmodern turn"—that frames such research as capable of understanding empirically "the complex and heterogeneous worlds emerging through new world orderings" (xxvii). This method allows for fine-grained analyses of genetic evidences' backstage machinations.

Clarke's (2005) approach proposes researchers use "meso-level analytic frameworks" such as "social worlds/arenas maps" (110). Social worlds and arena maps grant researchers a rich understanding of relationships or intersections between individuals, activities, technologies, and so forth. Another advantage of Clarke's method is that it assumes boundaries between concepts are porous. That is, researchers can see how actions, structures, and discourses spill into and onto one another. In the case of genetic testing, for instance, the analytic concept of site may include not only the scientific laboratory but also a specific nucleotide position located on a human gene. This method proves especially salient given that genetic evidences involve the coproduction of bodies, biologies, geographies, and technologies. Clarke pro-

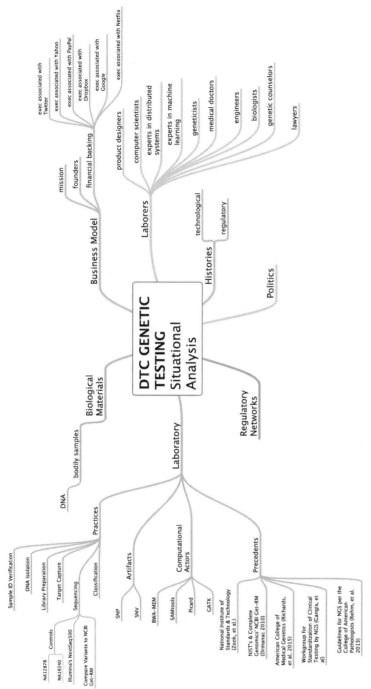

Figure 5.1 Early attempt at mapping direct-to-consumer genetic testing

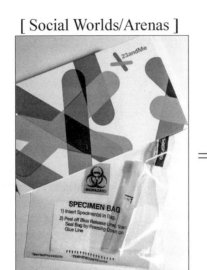

**[ Social Worlds/Arenas ]**

$=$

**[ Concepts ]**
Universes of discourse /
situations / identities /
commitments / shared ideologies /
primary activities / particular
sites / technologies / specialized
knowledges / more formal
organizations / going concerns /
entrepreneurs / mavericks /
segments/subworlds / reform
movements / bandwagons /
intersections / segmentations /
implicated actors and actants /
work objects / discourses

Figure 5.2 Clarke's conceptual toolbox (Clarke 2005, 112). 23andMe image from https://flic.kr/p/4pcvWf (image used by permission of Cedric Huesler).

vides a conceptual toolbox to aid researchers in becoming attuned to the particularities of certain social worlds/arenas: "These sensitizing concepts may be of help in creating social worlds/arenas maps, in locating the stories of particular interest vis-à-vis social worlds in your data, and in analysis" (112). Figure 5.2 is a visual rearticulation of the toolbox she includes in *Situational Analysis: Grounded Theory after the Postmodern Turn.*

Clarke (2005) does not intend for social worlds/arenas maps to render a theory of everything. Rather, by identifying overlap or intersections between concepts, situational maps help researchers decide which part of the situation deserves analytic attention. "As usual, we the researchers must delimit our stories to those that we can tell coherently. . . . It is highly unlikely that the final reports of a given research project, even one focused particularly on social worlds and arenas, will tell even all the 'big stories' framed by the social worlds/arenas map. Rather, the map should help you determine which stories to tell" (Clarke 2005, 111). The main assumption behind this chapter's methodological approach is that the direct-to-consumer genetic testing movement is actually not at all direct. Hidden in the shadows of direct-to-consumer genetic testing (i.e., Clarke's social world) is material-discursive labor (i.e., Clarke's concepts) of which consumers remain largely unaware even though they may use this information to make important decisions about their lifestyle or medical care. The following situational analyses of backstage methods for or shadow work involved in direct-to-consumer genetic sequencing—including "all analytically pertinent nonhuman (including technical) elements along with the human" (Clarke 2005, 63)—complicates politicized promises of precision in cancer care, medical empowerment, and individual autonomy.

## SITUATIONAL ANALYSES OF
## DIRECT-TO-CONSUMER GENETIC TESTING

I identified at least ten situational objects of study within direct-to-consumer genetic testing companies' texts, objects, human bodies, regulatory bodies, and human and nonhuman laborers (text box 5.1). Note how each of these situational objects of study are embedded in a host of other institutional and technological agents. It would be impossible, for example, to study the mission statements of genetic testing companies without also considering their business models and financial investors. It would be impossible to isolate and study regulatory decisions about genetic testing without understanding the complex roles of governmental agencies and their charter documents (including, e.g., the FDA; the Clinical Laboratory Improvement Amendments; the Federal Trade Commission; Health and Human Services; and public comments posted to "Optimizing Regulatory Oversight of Next Generation Sequencing Diagnostic Tests Public Workshop" on regulations.gov). According to Clarke (2005), a situational map "does not tell an analytic story but rather frames that story through mapping the broader situation as a whole and all the elements in it at a more general and abstract level" (137). In this next step, then, I map relationships between elements by identifying overlaps or intersections between situational concepts. In sum, analytic intersections between concepts are rich sites for understanding the backstage labor responsible for elevating genetic evidence to powerful and persuasive positions.

Clarke's (2005) conceptual toolbox (fig. 5.1) provides a list of twelve generic, but generative concepts, which I mobilized to develop a concept list specific to direct-to-consumer genetic testing. Each of these salient concepts is listed in text box 5.2. Some of the concepts in text box 5.2 are the result of coalescing several of Clarke's original concepts from figure 5.1. By way of example, for my purposes, I coalesced Clarke's identities, commitments, and specialized knowledges into one, overarching concept: universes of discourse.

In table 5.1, I provide definitions and examples for each of the study's concepts. In most cases, Clarke's (2005) actual definitions are used. In some

**Text box 5.1. Situational Objects of Study**

Direct-to-consumer companies' missions, business models, and financials / Direct-to-consumer companies' human laborers / Direct-to-consumer companies' published research and white papers / Direct-to-consumer companies' nonhuman laborers and labor (in vivo codes: assays, libraries, annotation and interpretation schemes, databases) as evidenced by direct-to-consumer companies' data sheets, direct-to-consumer companies' patents / Direct-to-consumer companies' informational materials / Regulatory decisions and deliberations about genetic testing in general and direct-to-consumer genetic testing specifically, as per the Food and Drug Administration, the Clinical Laboratory Improvement Amendments, the Federal Trade Commission, Health and Human Services, Secretary's Advisory Committee on Genetics, Health, and Society, results from relevant litigation, Genetics and Public Policy Center, Government Accountability Office, public comments posted to "Optimizing Regulatory Oversight of Next Generation Sequencing Diagnostic Tests Public Workshop" on regulations .gov (as of March 20, 2015) / Human consultant labor that assists genetic testing corporations with meeting the government's regulatory requirements for approval / Political movements for medical reform as per President Obama's "precision medicine initiative" / The landscape of competing genetic testing technologies (e.g., laboratory developed tests, next-generation sequencing) / Historical landscape of genetic testing techniques

---

**Text box 5.2. Salient Concepts for Situational Analysis of Direct-to-Consumer Genetic Testing**

universes of discourse (i.e., identities, commitments, specialized knowledges) / activities / sites / technologies / formal organizations / going concerns / entrepreneurs / reform movements / intersections / implicated actors and actants / boundary objects / discourses cases, however, definitions for concepts are modified versions of Clarke's so as to stay as close as possible to this study's situational context. I provide examples that operationalize each concept within specific methods for direct-to-consumer genetic testing at 23andMe and Color Genomics.

Mapping relationships and intersections between concepts identified in table 5.1 fosters interesting revelations about how 23andMe and Color Genomics attune themselves to bodies in flux. In the next section, I provide results from situational analyses of the following conceptual relationships.[9]

1. Technologies + Reform Movements + Going Concerns[10]
2. Discourses + Sites + Implicated Actors/Actants
3. Technologies + Entrepreneurs + Universe of Discourses + Implicated Actors/Actants

## ANALYSIS 1: INTERSECTIONS BETWEEN TECHNOLOGIES + REFORM MOVEMENTS + GOING CONCERNS

In genetic testing, technologies and reform movements intersect in revelatory ways. To date, most genetic scientists use next-generation genetic sequencing, which allows for sequencing larger data sets at a lower cost than ever before. According to Illumina, Inc. (a global company responsible for the technology used in almost 90 percent of the world's genetic sequencing), next-generation sequencing has "unprecedented throughput, scalability, and speed" that "enables researchers to study biological systems at a level never before possible" (Illumina 2016). Illumina boasts that their technological product "can deliver data output ranging from 300 kilobases up to 1 terabase in a single run" (Illumina 2016). Obama's Precision Medicine Initiative (one of this study's "reform movements") relies implicitly on Illumina and several other for-profit corporations whose technologies monopolize the genetic sequencing market. Many of these corporations are profiting quite handsomely from this "new era of data-based and more precise medical treatment" ("Fact Sheet," 2015) by circumventing hospitals and medical providers altogether and marketing directly to consumers. The at-home genetic testing kits available today, some of which are marketed as ancestry tracing, or what Kramer (2015) calls "a technology of belonging" (80), are direct-to-consumer products that rely on Illumina's technology.

Consumers concerned with individual autonomy and choice (one of this study's "going concerns") intersect with reform movements or political initiatives—initiatives whose going concerns are efficacy, regulation, and cost. Situational overlap between consumers and political initiatives further intersect with for-profit companies who provide the very technologies through

### Table 5.1 Concepts, Definitions, and Examples

| Concept | Definition | Examples |
|---------|-----------|----------|
| Universes of discourse | "Social worlds … and principal affiliative mechanisms through which people organize social life" (Clarke 2005, 46) | Computer science, product designer, genetics, biology, engineering, medical practice, genetic counseling, legal, capitalism, medicine |
| Activities | Human or nonhuman labor | Marketing, specific laboratory practices (e.g., DNA isolation, library preparation, classification, target capture); legislating/regulating; computing |
| Sites | A locatable space or place | Laboratory; court of law; human body; geographic locations; nucleotide positions on a gene; exomes |
| Technologies | An agent or actant that helps to organize work and/or affect activity | The gene; Illumina's NextSeq500; Control genes (NA12878; NA19240) |
| Formal organizations | A group of people with a particular disciplinary concern focused on resolving or investigating that concern | The National Institute of Standards and Technology; NIST; Complete Genomics; American College of Medical Genetics; Workgroup for Standardization of Clinical Testing by NGS; 23andMe, Inc.; Color Genomics, Inc. |
| Going concerns | "Assumptions about what activities are important and what will be done" (per Hughes 1971) | Privacy; accuracy; verifiability; sustainability; profitability |
| Entrepreneurs | Human actors who are "deeply committed and active individuals and cluster around the core of the social world and mobilize those around them" (Clarke 2005, 46) | Color Genomics's founders |

**Table 5.1 Continued**

| Concept | Definition | Examples |
|---|---|---|
| Reform movements | A social or political movement organized around a desire to change some aspect of medicine, health, technology, or society | Precision Medicine Initiative |
| Intersections | Overlap between one or more concepts | The overlap between sites and technologies (e.g., a single nucleotide position + target capturing) |
| Implicated actors and actants | "Actors and/or actants silenced or only discursively present— constructed by others for their own purposes" (Clarke 2005, 46) | Polymorphism; mutation; variation |
| Boundary objects | A human or object (material and processural) that "resides between social worlds" and is "ill structured," or has "interpretive flexibility" (per Star 2010) | Genetic reference materials; the gene itself |
| Discourses | "Modes of ordering the chaos of the world" (Foucault, quoted in Clarke 2005, 54) | Computational algorithms (e.g., HaploScore; BWA-MEM; SAMtools; Picard; GATK) |

which such going concerns may be resolved. The thread connecting each of these three analytic concepts (technologies, reform movements, going concerns)—that is, the thing that allows them to intersect and be in relationship—is reference material.

### WHAT IS REFERENCE MATERIAL?

*At the time that I write this, the genetic sequencing method that 23andMe conducts is called DNA profiling, or single nucleotide polymorphism (SNP) genotyping.[11] This method is a different and more affordable technique for genetic testing than sequencing an individual's whole genome. With this technique, a portion of an individual's DNA is compared with the DNA of known populations—or reference material. Reference materials are akin to a control group in a scientific experiment and are used during genetic testing as comparisons for individuals' genetic information.*

*The portion of a consumer's DNA that genetic scientists use for comparison is called a SNP (pronounced "snip"). When compared with SNPs from reference materials stored in a database, and after using algorithms for detecting matching patterns between the consumer's SNP and SNPs from reference materials, genetic scientists posit probabilities about an individual's genetic makeup. Genetic testing companies' technologies, concerns about profitability and accuracy, the desire to make medicine more precise, and consumers' choice and autonomy all rest on the richness of a genetic testing company's reference material database. Once SNPs from reference materials are collected and compared, scientists identify genetic markers that, based on these comparisons, appear to be correlated with a wide range of diseases—including some cancers.*

*Not every genetic testing company uses the same database of reference material, however. Color Genomics (2016) describes in a white paper published on their website that "every sequencing run contains two positive controls (NA12878 and NA19240) which have been recommended as reference material by the National Institute of Standards and Technology" (2). Whether other genetic testing companies are using these controls is another story. Aware of the unstandardized nature of reference materials and acknowledging that "the regulation of DNA tests … is complicated and in flux," the National Institute of Standards and Technology recently developed reference materials "that could be used by laboratories to determine whether their machines and software were properly analyzing a person's genetic blueprint, or genome" (Pear 2015). These standardized reference materials cost $450 a vial and include 10 micrograms of DNA from a woman of European ancestry who lives (or at one point lived) in Utah. The importance of reference material persists in the next two analyses.*

## ANALYSIS 2: INTERSECTIONS BETWEEN
## DISCOURSES + SITES + IMPLICATED ACTORS/ACTANTS

Genetic scientists locate and isolate a specific portion of an individual's genome for analysis and then use a unique, black-boxed discourse or algorithm (e.g., BWA-MEM, SAMtools, Picard, GATK) to detect similarities and differences between their reference material and the genetic information under analysis.[12] Unlike 23andMe's sequencing technique described above, which relies on detecting single nucleotide polymorphisms (SNPs), Color Genomics relies on exome sequencing. This method focuses on a different analytic site in a genome: the exome. Below I describe in greater detail each of these analytic concepts and the meaningfulness of the relationships and intersections between them. I conclude that genetic scientists' decisions about (*a*) which computational code they will use to perform computational analyses and (*b*) where, along the gene, they will direct their analytic gaze (SNPs vs. exons) ultimately affects how a genetic mutation is defined discursively.

### Discourses: GATK, HaploScore, and Computational Cut Making

According to Clarke (2005) discourses are "modes of ordering the chaos of the world" (54). In direct-to-consumer genetic testing one discourse relied on regularly for ordering the chaos of bodies in flux is the computational algorithm. In their white paper, Color Genomics (2016) describes that their "bioinformatics pipeline was built using well-established algorithms such as BWA-MEM, SAMtools, Picard and GATK" (1). On GATK's website (which stands for "genome analysis tool kit"), they boast: "Your plant has six copies of each chromosome? Bring it on" (GATK 2012). GATK relies on a command-line interface (versus a graphical user interface) compatible with Linux and OS X platforms. Direct-to-consumer genetic testing companies do, in fact, use different alignment algorithms and sequencing software. This is one reason why the same DNA can result in a very different set of alignments or mismatches between the source genetic material and the reference material to which it is compared.[13] Even the American College of Medical Genetics and Genomics published a series of standards and guidelines for interpreting genetic difference and similarity that recommend "the use of multiple software programs for sequence variant interpretation . . . because the different programs each have their own strengths and weaknesses, depending on the algorithm" (Richards et al. 2015, 5). Backstage biomedical discourses—in this case, algorithms and other computational code written for specific sequencing software—shape genetic evidences.

23andMe purportedly uses an algorithm called HaploScore. The "haplo" in HaploScore is a reference to haplotypes, which are clusters of tightly linked genes that are inherited from one parent. Efforts have been made to collaboratively map haplotypes toward an international and comprehensive collection of genetic sequencing data. Such a collection could be evidential grounds on which genetic scientists could devise a rich reference material database. The International HapMap Project, for example, is a collaboration between scientists in Canada, China, Japan, Nigeria, the United Kingdom, and the United States aimed at producing a publicly available database of haplotypes.

Computational code might then be written in such a way that an individual's genetic information could be compared with reference material from the HapMap, and differences between the two could be detected algorithmically.

To put it as simply as possible, algorithms are the result of computational code that, because of how it is written, can detect differences between reference material and the DNA splices under investigation. Computational methods of ordering the world (Clarke 2005) involve a two-stage process: The search stage, followed by an alignment stage. "The search stage finds regions in the genome that can potentially be homologous to the read. The alignment stage verifies these regions to check if they are indeed homologous. The alignment stage is usually more computationally intensive than the search stage and the time taken is directly proportional to the number of regions found in the search stage. Hence, the best strategy to a fast sequence mapping algorithm is to filter out as many candidate regions as possible before the alignment stage" (Misra et al. 2011, 190). Because of what they call a "dynamically changing genomic sequence," Iliopoulos et al. (2012) designed an algorithm that "takes into account ... replacement, insertions, deletions" (15). Based in part on filtering techniques, or computational cut making (Barad 2007, 115), these algorithms are a powerful discourse designed to make sense out of what is otherwise overwhelming informational chaos present in a small splice of a single chromosome.

Genetic scientists' difference machines (Brown 2014) are built, quite literally, to detect patterns of similarity and difference. A series of material and computational cuts must be made to the chromosome under study prior to running the code. The coding languages that make difference detection possible are not merely a way to render a priori differences visible. Rather, code is an act or performance of computational cut making; it is "a significant rhetorical component of textual creation" and "influences certain possibilities to become realized over others" (Brock 2012, 7, 5). If, as described in greater detail below, there is neither standard reference material nor standardized procedures by which genetic differences are computed, attention must be paid to the wide range of protocols and procedures by which genetic scientists make cuts. Attention must be paid to how computational cuts perform and produce difference. Now that readers have a sense of some of the discourses involved in computational cut making, the next section explores the intra-actional (Barad 2007) role of "sites" in determining genetic difference and similarity.

### Sites: Exomes

A very small portion of the human genome (approximately 1 percent) includes exons, which are a very specific sequence of nucleotides. Exons do a lot of important work in maintaining the human body's function and health. Once overlooked and characterized as junk DNA, scientists now understand that these nucleotides provide energy to cells, play a central role in one's metabolism, and provide important signals to cells about how to behave. Although exons account for only 1 percent of a person's genome, because they are so important to bodies' functioning and health, if there is a mutation anywhere along their sequence, the consequences are much more severe than when there are mutations in any other part of the genome. Genetic scientists have learned that by isolating and tracking the frequency of a particular nucleotide variation in the exome, one might gain a fuller understanding of how certain disorders, diseases, and other conditions are passed down from one generation to the next. To do that, scientists developed a method of genetic testing called exome sequencing.

Exome sequencing affords the isolation and identification of particular genetic variations that are thought to be associated with heritable diseases.[14] Variations in the same gene are called alleles (to remember this, it might be helpful to know that "allele" is a shortened version of "allelomorph," a Latin cognate of "alias," or "other form"). Scientists have begun to link claims about a person's increased risk for certain cancers with alleles in their exome. Scientists have made great strides in locating where, exactly, in the exome alleles present themselves. Moreover, they are able to say with some specificity which genes (if they contain certain mutations) may be linked with increased risk for certain cancers. In the case of breast and ovarian cancers, for example, genetic scientists have isolated somewhere between nineteen and twenty-five genes as potential culprits for harboring cancer-causing mutations. In response, scientists developed a technique for analytically targeting these specific genes, and engineers have helped such analyses along by designing technologies to accomplish sequencing at a much more rapid pace than ever before. Sequencing a single human exome requires anywhere from three to five terabytes of computational storage space. Exome sequencing is—quite literally—a big data project. What can ultimately be said about an individual's genetic risk hinges on where along the genome, or at which nucleotide position, researchers direct their analytic gaze. Now that I've explicated the role that computational discourses and sites (or nucleotide position) play in genetic sequencing, I will continue the analysis by explicating that which genetic scientists seek to delineate: polymorphism, genetic variation, and mutation. Under the rubric of Clarke's situational analysis method, I characterize these contributors as implicated actors and actants.

## Implicated Actors/Actants:
## Polymorphisms, Variations, Mutations

Above, I described 23andMe's use of SNPs, or single nucleotide polymorphisms. When genetic companies like Color Genomics analyze the exome, however, they do not use the SNP method. They use a method whereby single nucleotide variations, or SNVs, are detected. Single nucleotide variations earn their name because scientists have identified them in less than 1 percent of the reference material to which the consumer's genetic information is compared. Because their frequency is so rare, SNVs are considered "mutations." In contrast, polymorphisms (SNPs) earn their name when a variation is considered common in at least 1 percent of the population. Scientists use algorithms to identify SNVs. To do this, computational code is written to detect and match patterns of similarity and difference between the exome under analysis and the reference material. And yet, as described above, there is not (yet) a standard gene sequence, or reference material, to which all other genetic sequences are compared. What is considered "normal" or not-a-variation is a matter of frequency, therefore. There is no inherent biological or genetic difference between a SNP or a SNV (or mutation); these characterizations and all claims associated with them are a matter of frequency based on the laboratory's choice of reference material. Nelson (2008) explains it this way: "Algorithms and computational mathematics are used to analyze the samples and infer the individual's admixture of three or four statistically constituted categories—sub-Saharan African, Native American, East Asian, and European—according to the presence and frequency of specific genetic markers said to be predominate among, but importantly, not distinctive of, each of the original populations" (766). Genetic variation frequencies within reference populations change every day as scientists gather more and more reference data and as these data are packaged and commoditized differently by different laboratories.

Definitions for and delineations between SNP, SNV, and mutation are malleable at best and at worst, indeterminate. Consider that when a genetic variation is present that occurs in less than 1 percent of the reference population, scientists will classify that variation as a rare mutation. Yet, the same variation in a different time or place (or when compared to a different reference population) may actually confer resistance to a harmful biological or environmental agent. And because of natural selection, it is likely that greater than 1 percent of the population may, in fact, possess such a resistance-conferring genetic variation. Once that variation is present in greater than 1 percent of a population, scientists then go on to classify such a variation as a polymorphism—*not* a mutation. What would be categorized as a mutation in one time and at one geographical location might, therefore, be categorized a polymorphism in another time and place. The allele variation associated with sickle cell disease, for example, is a rare, life-threatening mutation in one time and place but confers resistance to malaria in another time and place; populations defined by the latter time and place may have survived, in part, because of this variation. Such a genetic variation is at once a life-threatening mutation and a life-saving polymorphism, depending on the time and place a population member inhabits. The sickle cell allele is but one example of how genetic variations—in particular, classifications for mutation versus polymorphism—involve discursive reductions of intra-acting bodies, time, places, and materials. Other examples of genetic sequencing's evidential malleability exist. TallBear's (2013) analysis, for instance, points to ways in which Native American DNA "is not simply naturally determined; it becomes manifest as scientists observe the movement of particular nucleotides via human bodies across time and space (between what is today Siberia/Asia and the Americas). The presence of such markers is then used to animate particular 'populations' and individuals and their tissues (both dead and living) as belonging to that identity category" (12). Nucleotide variations are made to matter because of the ways genetic scientists pattern-match such variations with other nucleotide variations from a particular geographic region. O'Rourke (2003), the former president of the American Association of Physical Anthropology, says it best: "Much of the uncertainty regarding evolutionary inferences of populations relates to the ephemeral nature of populations and the often arbitrary nature of population definitions. . . . This difficulty stems from the fluidity of individual and group identities in time and space. Individuals may change ethnic identities, and, hence, group membership, at will, complicating assumptions of demographic continuity over time" (104). Note here O'Rourke's acknowledgment of the fluid and ephemeral nature of population definitions. If population definitions or reference material don't stand still, how might that affect genetic scientists' assertions about similarity and difference? Recall that for Clarke (2005), implicated actors/actants are "only discursively present—constructed by others for their own purposes" (46). The genetic mutation, then, is the quintessential "implicated actor" in the practice of genetic sequencing.

In a way, direct-to-consumer genetic testing's focus on geographic space as having implications for what is defined as either mere polymorphic variation or life-threatening mutation has resulted in precisely the kind of thing Lefebvre (1974) warned us about: "Knowledge falls into a trap when it makes

representations of space the basis for the study of 'life,' for in doing so it reduces lived experience" (230). Here again, we see the importance of reference
material in genetic testing companies' computational backstage. Reference
materials are the connecting thread between each of these seemingly dispa-
rate analytic concepts.[15] Reference materials stabilize (for now) how a population is defined, how geographies are mapped, and the claims that can be
made about what bodies are or will be.

### ANALYSIS 3: INTERSECTIONS BETWEEN UNIVERSES OF DISCOURSES + ENTREPRENEURS + TECHNOLOGIES + IMPLICATED ACTORS/ACTANTS

In the above situational map, "universes of discourses," defined by Clarke
(2005) as "social worlds . . . and principal affiliative mechanisms through
which people organize social life" (46), are meant to draw researchers' attention to all the things that bear up and make possible that which we come to
characterize as evidence. I identified each of the following as its own discourse
universe: computer science / product design / genetics / biology / engineering / medical practice / genetic counseling / legal. The "convergence[s] between different previously differentiated branches of technology," as Braidotti
(2007) argues, "are equally co-present in driving home the spectacular effects
of contemporary technological transformations" (67). Converging disciplines
toward the accomplishment of some "euphoric celebration of new technologies" (Braidotti 2007, 66) would seem promising and potentially revolution-
ary, but the "gravitational pull of old and established values" (66) between
each of these discourse universes complicates that euphoria. While medical
precision is a kind of mandate in the United States, the human and nonhuman labor that makes such a technoscientific promise possible consists
mostly of inexact, computational rhetorics: Splicing. Cutting. Pattern matching. As demonstrated in analysis number 2 above, the very means by which
genetic variations are categorized as mutation or mere polymorphism is a
discursive construction that results from algorithmic pattern matching and
statistical calculations of frequency.

When entrepreneurs are added to the network of intra-acting discourse
universes identified above, the rhetorical act of managing risks associated
with bodies in flux are made all the more complex. *Bloomberg Business* reports that,

> along with Khosla [Ventures] and [Laurene Powell] Jobs [Steve Jobs's
> widow], Color Genomics is backed by venture capital investment firm

Formation 8, as well as BlackRock Inc. co-founder Susan Wagner and Cisco System Inc.'s Chief Technology Officer Padmasree Warrior. It's also advised by Mary-Claire King, the geneticist who discovered the BRCA1 gene.

Based in Burlingame, California, Color Genomics is staffed with a mix of biologists and computer scientists, along with engineers who previously worked at Twitter Inc., Google Inc. and LinkedIn Corp. (Chen 2015, n.p.)

The majority of Color Genomics' financial backers and scientific team are experts from information and communication technology industries. Similarly, Google is a major financial backer of 23andMe. Nowotny (2007) and Parry (2013) challenge readers to consider effects of technoscientific partnerships after they have entered spheres of commodification. Parry, in particular, argues that direct-to-consumer genetic companies are "commoditizing material evidence of your latent future" (161). Consumers' lack of understanding about how, exactly, material-discursive evidences are computed and commoditized may mean they are ill-equipped to make decisions about how their bioinformation is (or ought to be) valued—both monetarily and medically.

Investigating the backstage technological details of how genetic evidences are computed is especially necessary not just because of how evidences are commoditized and sold to otherwise healthy individuals (what Pender [2012] calls the "pre-ill"), but also because such evidences are often accompanied by narratives of individualism, empowerment, and choice. Overlap between universes of discourses, entrepreneurs, and technologies elevate quotidian biological snapshots and processes from benign concurrent engineerings (cf. Lee et al. 2013) to economically viable forms of evidence. Their overlap is not merely epiphenomenal to resultant arguments about ancestry, genetic risk, and medical vulnerability. Taken together, their overlap implicates precision medicine's central actor: the genetic mutation. How matter is made to mean in genetic science attunes experts and everyday citizens alike to bodies in flux in potentially precarious ways.

To the network of genetic evidential coproduction, entrepreneurs contribute not just their technological skill and business acumen but also overarching concerns about and an interest in profitability. Persuasive marketing materials frame at-home genetic tests as a way of truly knowing ourselves. Genetic testing options geared toward women are framed as a choice or a right (and in today's political climate, a woman's choice or right to take control of her body is a highly valued commodity). Other arguments frame the decision to perform at-home genetic testing as more than mere choice, but an actual responsibility since "the benefits to future generations could be enormous" (Karen Rothenberg, quoted in Happe 2013, 59).

Implicit in the Precision Medicine Initiative and in direct-to-consumer genetic testing companies' marketing practices are narratives that promise not only individual benefit but also contributions to a greater good. Such narratives might best be characterized as what Wendy Brown (2015) terms "*omnes et signulatim*"—"all and each—power exercised through massification and isolation" (71). It is indeed true that when a consumer or patient provides her genetic information (usually in the form of a saliva or blood sample), that information can then become part of the reference material database to which future SNPs or SNVs are pattern matched. Building such a database is important for genetic testing corporations since they often use claims about the richness of their reference material as a marketing tactic. Under the rubric of precision medicine, you, too, can be a biomedical entrepreneur: possessing and contributing your unique genetic makeup confirms your value as human capital in a more precise and personalized care network.[16]

Although the White House's Precision Medicine Initiative does not explicitly incorporate at-home genetic testing kits in its promise of more precise care, the situational analyses above indicate that there is an economic and technoscientific partnership between the initiative and Illumina—one of (if not the only) major technoscientific corporations responsible for the majority of genetic testing technology. As biomedicine moves from evidence-based medicine toward a precision medicine model, we should anticipate not only that patients are now characterized as consumers, but also that, as Murray and Steinberg (2015) argue, "production and consumption" will "become indistinguishable" (129). More to the point: we should anticipate that results from our genetic testing will be incorporated automatically into a single, robust reference material database funded by the government, monitored by for-profit corporations, and standardized by bureaucratic, regulatory networks made up of experts from each of the aforementioned universes of discourse. Within such a network of evidential coproduction, "spaces of ambiguity are collapsed and supplanted by the systemic 'knowledge' of predictive rationality, risk-management, securitization, and then handed over to a cadre of 'expert' service providers in the management of one's own livingness" (Murray and Steinberg 2015, 135). Importantly, the individual and collective power of each of these contributors to a network of genetic evidential production is still only as good as its reference material. In other words, that which both allows each of the above contributors to be in evidential relationship and makes possible the collapse of ambiguity or the kind of "terribly difficult state of mind" brought about by medical uncertainty (Dahl 2016) is reference material. What, then, can rhetorical theory teach us about how genetic materials in general and reference material in particular are elevated to positions of evidential power?

## UNDERSTANDING REFERENCE MATERIALS
## AS BOUNDARY OBJECTS

According to Clarke (2005), studying boundary objects "can be an important pathway into often complicated situations" (51). Drawing on Star and Griesemer (1989), Clarke defines a boundary object as either a human or nonhuman thing that "exist(s) at junctures where varied social worlds meet in an arena of mutual concern" (50). For Derkatch (2008), because boundary objects are rhetorically mobile they enable research across dissimilar fields and can be used strategically, even if unconsciously, to advance certain argumentative ends.[17] Ideologically and practically malleable (yet robust), boundary objects help people do work—they help us "do things with things" (Barnett and Boyle 2016). Star (2010) clarifies that to be concerned with a boundary object is to investigate "how practices structure, and language emerge, for doing things together" (602). Boundaries are a "shared space" where "here and there are confounded" (Star 2010, 602–3). I argue that in direct-to-consumer genetic testing, reference materials are boundary objects.

Examining intra-actions (Barad 2007) between each of the above phenomena yields a richer understanding of the role boundary objects play in direct-to-consumer genetic sequencing. When genetic scientists translate results from intra-acting phenomena into something that resembles actionable evidence, they do so based on comparisons to *reference material*. Reference material includes genetic information from genes and bodies that have been analyzed previously. The ontological intra-actional yield (of technologies, actants, actors, discourses, sites, activities, etc.) is compared to a boundary object (which is, as well, a result of ontological intra-actions, but from an earlier time), and from those comparisons evidential inferences are made. Mapping and analyzing the ontological collision of assays, algorithms, polymorphisms, and other phenomena tells a larger story about the gene as a coconstituted site (Haraway 1997) and demonstrates the rhetorical power of reference material.

Boundary objects (such as reference materials) help people do things with things because they fill the gap or space once imagined as a boundary. They are, according to Star (2010), "n-dimensional" (603). Boundary work describes the performance of gap filling. Such a performance is rhetorical; rigid rules and finite divisions no longer hold. In a world where all is flux, situational elements simply bleed (Edbauer 2005), and biological indeterminacies abound, reference materials are the quintessential boundary object. Reference materials are coproduced phenomena that both compute and are computed from other coproduced phenomena. Results from genetic sequencing "can only be validated and interpreted in light of the results of others" (Kramer 2015, 85). Reference materials, therefore, move us out of ambiguity and indeterminacy toward probabilities of a particular corporeal future. The rhetorical mechanism or argumentative substrate by which such a move is made successful is what I will now refer to as a boundary infrastructure.

## REFERENCE MATERIALS' RHETORICAL INFRASTRUCTURE

Although it receives less attention than "boundary object," Star's (2010) "boundary infrastructure" is useful here for explaining how each of the above phenomena intra-act (Barad 2007) and make it possible to attune (Rickert 2013) to bodies in flux. For Star, boundary infrastructures are rhetorically mobile in that they, regardless of their accuracy in specific situations, are useful to a wide range of stakeholders. Star illustrates boundary infrastructures by invoking David Ferrier's research, which, astonishingly to her, was hugely successful despite the fact that it made claims about the human brain based only on sketches of a monkey's brain. Says Star (2010), "Ferrier took the expedient step of simply taking the monkey map and transposing the circles marking functional areas directly onto the human brain sketch" (608). Skeptical that such a move could possibly provide anything useful, Star likens Ferrier's "tacking back-and-forth" (613) between one thing and another to "taking a map of the Paris subway and superimposing it on Cleveland, and using it to talk about traveling around Cleveland, reasoning that all large cities essentially have the same sort of transportation infrastructure" (608). Star determines that the reason Ferrier's map tacking was effective is because the resulting evidence only needed to "serve as the basis for conversation, for sharing data, for pointing to things—without actually demarcating any real territory" (608). In other words, the resulting evidence need only help people do things with things.

This chapter asserts that backstage computational methods for attuning genetically make up a powerful, predictive boundary infrastructure. Possibilities for future action (whether such action involves lifestyle changes or preventative surgeries) are based on backstage computational practices. These backstage computations are the intra-actional yield of a network of human and nonhuman things. Discursive boundaries between variation, polymorphism, or mutation are based on frequency calculations of data amassed from algorithmic cut making. Results from genetic sequencing create conversation and foster further data sharing but may not actually "demarcate any real territory" (Star 2010, 608). The fact that genetic sequencing may not "demarcate any real territory" is likely why 23andMe includes the following disclaimer on their website: "Our tests can be used to determine carrier status in adults …, but cannot determine if you have two copies of the genetic variant. Each test is most relevant for people of certain ethnicities. The tests are not intended to diagnose a disease, or tell you anything about your risk for developing a disease in the future. On their own, carrier status tests are not intended to tell you anything about the health of your fetus, or your newborn child's risk of developing a particular disease later in life." The fact that genetic sequencing may not "demarcate any real territory" is also why, as Kramer (2015) states, "some genetic genealogy spokespersons are also quick to refute the idea that genetic information can tell the 'full story'" (88).

The material-discursive labor required to elevate bioinformation to evidentiary status is not epiphenomenal to arguments about ancestry and/or genetic risk. Haraway (1997) asserted some time ago that genes are "material-semiotic objects of knowledge" that are "forged by heterogeneous practices in the furnaces of technoscience" (129). Analyses above describe some of the fodder from which such furnaces are fueled. As Jasanoff (2004) argues, "What happens in science and technology today is interwoven with issues of meaning, values, and power in ways that demand sustained critical inquiry" (29). In what follows, I posit several implications for what we now know about the backstage boundary work that makes possible computational analyses of genetic evidence.

### EVIDENTIARY SHADOW WORK IN GENETIC TESTING

Costs associated with evidential empowerment, precision, and personalized medicine are made invisible when consumers are encouraged through marketing and politicized promises of precision medicine to believe that "knowledge—or at least prospective knowledge—of one's bodily fate (e.g., predisposition to disease, hypersensitivity to allergens, and propensity to weight gain) is … a new type of commodity that, it is argued, will afford them, in keeping with the tenets of neoliberalism, unprecedented levels of personal autonomy in health care" (Parry 2013, 158). Cultural values of personal autonomy, empowerment, and choice are central to the success of direct-to-consumer genetic testing companies like 23andMe and Color Genomics. Several assumptions are implicit in how genetic tests are marketed as evidences that grant consumers and patients individual autonomy, empowerment, and choice. Parthasarathy (2014) argues that "the tantalizing prospect of genetic testing as a tool of empowerment rests on four key assumptions: that the information generated by this technology is accurate, easily understood, and benign; that the information produced is similarly empowering regardless of its utility; that it will have similar meaning and consequences regardless of the demographics of the user; and that offering this information directly to the end user will allow her to become sufficiently expert to make independent decisions about her life" (94). In this chapter, I have complicated each of these assumptions by detailing methods with which genetic evidences construct corporeal futures—in particular, the deployment of a contingent, nonstandardized boundary object: genetic reference material. Moreover, such backstage methods hinge on nonstandardized computational techniques for evidential cut making. In sum, direct-to-consumer genetic sequencing involves the act of tacking back and forth between "ill structured and well structured aspects" (Star 2010, 601).

Genetic sequencing is a rhetorical performance that involves computing the probability of risk by using algorithms that detect similarity and difference. Probabilities of risk are grounds on which conversations can be had about the future of a body in flux. Typically, these conversations are framed by using empowerment narratives (see also Lippman's [1991] "geneticization" and King's [1995] "invisible hand of individual choice"). To what degree does the act of revealing direct-to-consumer corporations' computational methods for evidential cut making pose the possibility of rescuing us from the cost of such narratives, then? To what degree do algorithms black-box powerful sociopolitical, economic, and biotechnoscientific assumptions that shape computational cut-making practices? Regardless of how the question is framed, it is clear that evidential attunement is never a value free, apolitical act—despite claims in support of genetic testing's "rationality and objectivity" (Kramer 2015, 86).

One of the constructs on which this book's analytic foci are predicated—Illich's (1981) shadow work—explains the unpaid labor associated with making particular goods and services possible. Given the era in which he was writing, Illich was concerned mostly with the kind of unpaid labor characteristic of industrialized economies. However, there is some alignment between industrial-age shadow work and the kind of invisible labor characteristic of today's information age. Illich says: "I call this complement to wage labor 'shadow work.' It comprises most housework women do in their homes and apartments, the activities connected with shopping, most of the homework of students cramming for exams, the toil expended commuting to and from the job. It includes the stress of forced consumption, the tedious and regimented surrender to therapists, compliance with bureaucrats, the preparation for work to which one is compelled, and many of the activities usually labeled 'family life'" (100). According to Illich, this labor is "hidden by the industrial-age ideology"—not "subsistence activity" but shadow in that it is a "unique form of bondage" characteristic of "*homo economicus*" (100). Illich's claims about industrial societies' shadow work extend productively onto the kinds of backstage computational labor characteristic of an information economy. There is, after all, a good deal of invisible,[18] material-discursive toil that undergirds an information—and by extension, a bioinformational—economy. From Apple's Foxconn to the human laborers responsible for moderating content on Facebook, a host of computational rhetorics support or make possible end-user information consumption. Frequently, this labor is concealed not just by geographic distance but also because effective information architecture requires black-boxing the very means by which information is made consumable.

In the case of direct-to-consumer genetic sequencing, the shadow work is abundant: political promises of precision that carry with them the implicit fear that current methods are imprecise; entrepreneurial partnerships between seemingly otherwise incongruent discourse universes; the discursive and computational enactments of what counts as a mutation and how population boundaries will be defined (and the effects thereof on vulnerable populations); discourses whose computational algorithms for detecting difference and similarity are a result of coding practices and databases that are commoditized and deployed differently across time, space, and markets; and finally, the fear of disease and our subsequent desire for managing risks associated with living in a body in flux.[19]

It is tempting to eschew implications of how *homo oeconomicus* is bound up in scientific and medical progress and focus instead on seemingly benign computational methods of evidentiary production and medical precision. It is tempting to hang our hat simply on celebrations of technoscientific advances for detecting and treating cancer. Lauding the brilliance of technoscientific partnerships in sequencing efforts, Lee et al. (2013) argue that genetic research "is not simple science," but requires "the development of ingenious technologies by people with highly evolved engineering skills" (44). This chapter shifts our analytic gaze for a moment off of genetic sequencing's "ingenious technologies" and expert scientists' "highly evolved engineering skills" (Lee et al. 2013, 44) to account for the computational shadow work that orchestrates probabilistic predictions for "divining one's fate" (Parry 2013, 162).

I am reluctant to characterize computational methods for attuning evidentially as unscrupulous. But I do see a need for constant critical attention to how "all technologies have ... strong 'bio-power' effect[s]" that "affect bodies and immerse them in social relations of power, inclusion and exclusion" (Braidotti 2007, 67). As Pender (2012) argues, "For all of its scientific and technological advances, biomedicine continues to be an exclusionary enterprise that too often prioritizes corporate interests, leaving the health care needs of many unmet" (339). The biopower of genetic science is perhaps best illustrated in TallBear's (2013) analysis of DNA testing's precarious implications for Native American populations seeking sovereignty. TallBear makes the case that "genetics discourse can be used to 'other,' that is to represent some living human beings as not normative, as the sources of the raw materials of science, as the ancient, remote, less evolved, less enlightened ancestors of more modern living people" (202). TallBear states concern about "the power of DNA evidence to constitute history and identity in ways that risk indigenous land and governance rights" (203). Where we see biopower, then, we will find Illichian shadow work. This is to say nothing of how, under the guise of biological facticity (see Kramer 2015, 99), genetic testing as a way of attuning to bodies in flux reifies racist ideologies. It's also not within the scope of this chapter to attend to concerns about personal privacy that have emerged in this new era of precision medicine. Nevertheless, I hope that the above critical methodological unmaskings (Miller 2010) help to continue conversations about the material-discursive foundations of Illichian shadow work in genetic science.[20]

Taking to be true Scott's (2006) argument that, "despite its futility, the desire to predict, control, and avoid risk is still with us" (121), it behooves us to pause and consider the backstage computational labor involved in predicting, controlling, and avoiding risk. Before purchasing and simultaneously selling information about themselves, patients-turned-consumers-turned-reference material–turned-patients might do well to understand (if not inquire about) the nature of a particular laboratory's methods for genetic sequencing. Some of this information is available on the genetic testing company's website. But even I had to confirm what I'd learned about contemporary genetic testing methods (sussed out through companies' white papers, patent documents, and affiliated researchers' publications) with a key informant who is a licensed genetic counselor. Consumers also ought to be aware that their evidences will become part of future databases to which others' genetic information will be compared. Some refer to this as "biopiracy" or "biocolonialism" (TallBear 2013, 192–93). Consumers might choose, therefore, to read carefully a genetic testing company's biobanking consent documents. Beware, too, of the "evangelical aspect" to genetic testing—specifically: "Anybody's test results could have meaning for somebody else," which means that "it is always in the interest of those who have been tested to encourage others to be tested because with more comprehensive databases comes the increased possibility of a more nuanced interpretation of results" (Kramer 2015, 89). These examples represent only some of the shadow work now associated with computing evidence in genetic science.

Finally, I hope to have demonstrated that there is nothing more individualized, personal, or precise about attuning genetically to a body in flux. Computed evidences resultant from direct-to-consumer genetic testing methods rely on the same algorithmic, enthymematic rhetorics described in previous chapters. Chapter 3 theorized probability as *poesis* and described how attuning statistically involved enthymematic reasoning; chapter 4 described evidential synthesis as a matter of sifting systematically and rhetorically through that which would or would not count. This chapter details similar acts of evidential cut making and syntheses of large data sets in terms of rhetorical computation and boundary work. Genetic scientists synthesize evidences by partnering with computational rhetorics to cut, map tack, and pattern match. Such human and nonhuman partnerships and rhetorical performances are ways of attuning to evidential signal in a sea of informational noise. Cutting-edge, direct-to-consumer genetic testing companies may employ next-generation sequencing technologies. But even next-generation sequencing technologies' evidential yield hinges on rhetorical moves that are characteristic of pre- "precision medicine": specifically, freezing in time and place that which is presently known but is also, at present, now past; and working with rhetoric's algorithms to compute from genetic input a probabilistic prediction of that which, ultimately, cannot be predicted. In this sense, all rhetoric is, indeed, computational and all computation is rhetoric.

Both original genetic and reference materials are the result of intra-actions between geographical location, inherited genetic material, environmental contributors, economics, random mutations, epigenetics, and so on. To help make more transparent the conditions of and contributors to evidential cut making and practices of tacking back and forth between what is and cannot yet be known, we need an ethic of care that accounts for how bodies are, indeed, in perpetual flux. In the next and final chapter, I draw on findings from each of the previous chapters to frame medical practice as *phronesis*. In so doing, I hope to lay the groundwork for an ethic of care that is attuned to the inevitability of change over time—the inevitability of bodies in flux. I propose an ethic of care that is attuned to persons who are unaware, uninterested, or undereducated about how bodies (especially their genetic materials) are a result of previous and ongoing intra-actions. I propose an ethic of care that is attuned to how possibilities for future action are the result of coconstructed evidences. I propose an ethic of care that is mindful of hazards associated with managing risk, and can, as Alaimo (2008) puts it, "contend with . . . realities in which 'human' and 'environment' can by no means be considered as separate." Such an ethic of care demands attention to consequences of "environmental health, environmental justice, the traffic in toxins, and genetic engineering, to name a few" (Alaimo 2008, 239). I propose an ethic of care not as a normative, moral stance on what is right or wrong, but as a way of being (a body) in the world that embraces complexity and contingency over time and in space—an ethic that does not deny the "ambiguities of reality and the precariousness of human life" (Murray and Steinberg 2015, 135).

# 6. DWELLING WITH DISEASE

*The world is devious rather than dappled, too complex to*
*fit neatly into any of our models, theories, or explanations ... everything*
*is connected to everything else, even if in ways which often elude us and*
*may in fact remain forever beyond our grasp.*
Evelyn Fox Keller, *Making Sense of Life*

*We need to learn to think differently about ourselves and our*
*systems of values, starting with adequate cartographies of our embedded*
*and embodied positions.*
Rosi Braidotti, "Feminist Epistemology after Postmodernism"

*Disease is the corporeal effect of embodied social relations.*
Kelly E. Happe, *The Material Gene*

I began this book by asserting that defining and diagnosing disease is a kind of quixotic empiricism. In each chapter, I've tried to unpack such a paradox by describing biomedical evidences as material and methodical attunements to bodies—bodies in perpetual flux. In chapter 2, I described how visualizing evidence involves "vectors of material and discursive force" (Rickert [2013], 90; e.g., stains, slides, and scopes in the pathology laboratory) that, over time, evince the chaos of cancer. I made the case that navigating corporeal flux, especially at the cellular level, is an act of dwelling kairotically. In practice, dwelling kairotically requires the acknowledgment that medical decisions hinge on "workable or probable truths in situations lacking certainty" and "include and transcend human doing" (Rickert 2013, 81, 83).

Chapter 3 presented findings from a case study of evidential assessment during FDA pharmaceutical hearings. I described how, when assessing survival data, medical professionals rely on a chain of enthymematic premises (e.g., hazard rates, confidence intervals, effect size, and $p$ values) that "bring the world into rhetorical performance" (Rickert 2013, xviii). Since, according to Barad (2007), "measurement resolves the indeterminacy" (280), I borrowed Rickert's (2013) assumptions about the "stitchwork of material, practical, and discursive relations" in order to unpack how inferential statistical analysis does rhetorical work (93). Understanding evidential assessment as a form of enthymematic reasoning might lay the groundwork for greater reliance on alternative methods for attuning to different forms of survival data—

methods that capture the complexity of dwelling with cancer in ways that might resist quantification.

In chapter 4, I crafted an innovative analytic framework with which to understand the behind-the-scenes evidential synthesis labor employed by medical professionals. In particular, Toulmin's (2003) model for argumentation helped me to identify argumentative parts of speech within three Cochrane Systematic Reviews (CSRs), while modifications to stasis theory accounted for the rhetorical reasoning behind why more evidence was excluded than included in each CSR. Understanding evidential synthesis as an inherently rhetorical act that involves weighing and sifting data toward some final, generalizable claim yields a call to action: We need more cross-disciplinary collaborations among rhetoricians, technical communicators, and medical professionals. Such collaborations might help resolve procedural sticking points, resist conceptual cul-de-sacs, and sanction the validity of what Fleck calls "pluricentric collectives with different gravity centers and degrees of closure" (quoted in Peine 2011, 503). I hope, too, that this chapter demonstrates the value of rhetorical theory in practice—or what Fahnestock and Secor (1988) call "an instrument capable of performing … intricate analysis" (427).

Finally, in chapter 5 I described the vitality of reference materials in genetic scientists' algorithmic computation of corporeal differences—differences that may, in fact, under- or overemphasize the probability of a genetic mutation. I argued that the human and computational partnerships that emerge during genetic testing are, indeed, effective methods for attuning to evidential signals in a sea of informational noise; but evidential computation in genetic testing flattens if not silences intra-actions (Barad 2007) between geography, socioeconomics, and environment, all of which affect human health. I concluded by asking: To what degree do genetic testing's methods black-box powerful sociopolitical, economic, and biotechnoscientific assumptions that ultimately end up shaping scientists' computational cut-making practices?

On the whole, I have made the case that attunement practices in the biomedical backstage are not and can never be free from that which scientists seek to isolate and exclude as contributors to human health. Moreover, it is possible that scientists' attempts at isolating bodies from flux create, at best, unrealistic expectations and, at worst, undesirable care practices. Aside from the difficulty associated with attuning to fluctuating differences among individuals, populations, humans, things, this, and that are a host of other reasons for the indeterminacy inherent in cancer care. There is a lifetime of intellectual space left for ongoing investigations of such differences and difficulties. For now, however, at least three theoretical and practical propositions can be gleaned from this book's investigations of the biomedical backstage and all the ways medical and scientific professionals assemble evidential worlds from bodies in constant flux: (1) evidences result from rhetorical attunements; (2) methods matter; and (3) biomedical practice (not just health) is relational.

### EVIDENCES RESULT FROM RHETORICAL ATTUNEMENTS

Evincing bodies in flux requires a "constellation of abilities" (Vee 2010, 3); among these is rhetorical skill. In medical practice, rhetoric is a material-discursive performance that involves dissecting corporeal differences and similarities into manageable bits and bytes. Rhetoric is a material-discursive act of designing and deploying algorithmic protocols capable of predicting and communicating about possibility. Rhetorical attunements locate, find, and place (Rickert 2013) the inescapable entanglements, intra-actions (Barad 2007), and coimmersions that make what *is* (Bohm 1981). Doing medicine is a matter of rhetorical attunement. This book demonstrates that rhetorical attunement in contemporary biomedical practice requires dwelling kairotically (chap. 2), reasoning enthymematically (chap. 3), constantly critiquing the infrastructures and standards by which care is provided (chap. 4), and making computational cuts (chap. 5).

My analyses suggest that medical evidences perform the world *as it was* at a particular time and in a particular place. That is, evidences are not a priori articulations of what is but, rather, the result of a methodical, systematic performance of what *was*. To evince is to curate freeze-framed sociopolitical ideologies, matter, movement, and time. The degree to which we should rely on predictions of *what will be* hinges on how well we understand how *what is* came to be. In biomedical practice, claims about what is, was, and will be are enmeshed in methodological matter(s). When competing claims collide regarding what is and what was (as they did during cancer-care deliberations and in public policy hearings, CSRs, and genetic sequencing), backstage methods for attuning help to animate certain claims' probabilistic possibility.

One backstage method for attuning and thereby evincing cancer is enthymematic reasoning. Enthymemes are heuristics. They rely on algorithms and "proceduracy" (Vee 2010) to invent arguments about a body in flux. Even as enthymemes evince local phenomena (Brock 2014), they also constrain. The very population-based premise on which many evidential enthymemes in medical practice hinge may reveal one thing while simultaneously concealing another. In fact, I would argue that contemporary biomedicine's greatest challenge is the tension that arises when medical professionals reason en-thymematically about individual or local decisions by using population-based premises.

While on the one hand we know that population-based premises flatten if not sterilize localized experiences, on the other hand, population-based premises for localized decision making saves lives. Collins and Pinch (2008) put it this way:

> If we know one thing with near certainty, it is that the physical world, not to mention the body, will never be entirely understood at the level of detailed causal interactions—in the case of the body, the interactions between cells, chemical messengers, electrical pathways, and thoughts. Nevertheless, we have to hope for more transitions from PAT [popula-tion average testing] to SIC [specific individual cases]. We have to hope for this or we have to embrace an entirely different kind of society where reason is no longer a dominant value, and that is a society that, if we thought about it hard, we would realize we would not like: it would be a society in which, though population statistics for fatalities would no longer work as an argument for universal vaccination, they would also lose their force for seat-belt enforcement, for limiting the use of sport-utility vehicles, for limiting the distribution of guns, for cutting green-house emissions, and for reducing smoking in public places. (219–20)

Despite epideictic monikers like "evidence based," "next generation," and "precision," contemporary biomedical practice is inescapably enthymema-tic. It is tempting to disparage enthymematic reasoning for the ways it flat-tens and sterilizes localized experiences, but enthymemes only ever promise probabilistic possibility. They have never promised proof: "The person who argues from an enthymeme is [usually] not trying to *prove* a proposition" (Hairston 1986, 76). Recognizing that enthymematic reasoning lies at the heart of biomedical practice opens up potential for moving beyond epideictic rhetorics of praise or blame in medical practice and embracing the possibility of attuning to other sources of suasive evidential premises. Rhetoricians and technical communicators are uniquely positioned to contribute their exper-tise in enthymematic evidential attunement, even (and especially) with data that resist quantification or with data that lend support for arguments that do not seek to "*prove* a proposition" (Hairston 1986, 76).

## METHODS MATTER

Methods for attuning to bodies in flux materially make meaningful that which *was* at a particular time and place. Methods for mattering in evidence-based medicine are required to be systematic and transparent. Biomedicine's methodological transparency is thought to strip away the possibility of extrahuman and human error or interference and, perhaps, loan medical practice a sense of epistemic impersonality. However, in each case described in chapters 2–5, methods are bound up in and coconstructed alongside definitions for and diagnoses of disease. Intra-actions between material phenomena (e.g., cells, scopes, and stains) are premises on which prognostic potentiality or probability is calculated. Probabilistic estimates make and shape (*poesis*) how matter comes to matter. Seemingly benign criteria for assessing evidences have and do exert agencies. Computer algorithms exert suasive influence. Syntheses require cut making. Sequencing requires map tacking. These methods *matter*. Technologies do not merely intervene on illness or mediate care; biomedical technologies and care are mutually constitutive.

The idea that our bodies go on doing what they do long before we know to evidence them is not new. In 1932, Wells and Huxley described, "we are all cell communities ... and these cells ... can behave with remarkable individuality and independence" (quoted in J. Brown 2015, 326). Key to my argument, though, is that biomedicine's methods for attuning make meaningful our bodies' material processes. Methods, therefore, evidence; but things do, indeed, do. Evidence-based medicine, while methodologically systematic, cannot avoid matter's mattering. Barad (2003) issued a call for understanding "*how the body's materiality ... and other material forces actively matter to the process of materialization*" (809; italics in original). This book affirms that because matter persists at mattering, biomedical evidences cannot be anything but coconstructed phenomena.

### CARE IS RELATIONAL

Thus far, I have established that in the shadows of medical precision and so-called scientific progress are human, nonhuman, and extrahuman actors whose discreet labor makes possible the very evidences on which medical indeterminacy is navigated. Each chapter has mapped how such labor emerges through intra-actions and relationships between human, nonhuman, and extrahuman actors. And yet, "well-being is always in flux" (Atkinson et al. 2015, 77). Boundaries between time, place, patient, provider, and other contributors to a culture of health and well-being are messy and muddied. Such messy and muddied boundaries condition and assemble available means for "lively relationalities of becoming" (Barad 2007, 393). Coming to terms with lively relationalities of becoming requires attunement not only to bioinformational evidences but also to that which threatens such relationalities: biopower (Braidotti 2007). Under the rubric of biopower, cells are at risk of colonization. Biological materials are at risk of commoditization. Bodies are at risk of exploitation.

As I write this, the city of Flint, Michigan, continues to poison its citizens (many of whom are African American) with lead-laced water. As local, state, and federal officials seek to off-load responsibility onto nonhuman and biological actors (i.e., corroded pipes, bacteria), we see that our transcorporeal condition in general and "toxic bodies," in particular, "insist that environmentalism, human health, and social justice cannot be severed" (Alaimo 2008, 262). To argue that health is relational, therefore, is not enough. Were it enough, corroded pipes and bacteria would suffice as scapegoats for the national disaster that is Flint, Michigan. Care—not just health—is relational. Care extends well-being beyond the individual and exposes our "readiness to respond (a response-ability) that precedes both desire and will" (Davis 2005, 200); it requires us to acknowledge that healthist discourse is, as Bennett (2010) might argue, a kind of "Kantian morality" that forces some humans "to suffer because they do not conform to a particular (Euro-American, bourgeois, theocentric, or other) model of personhood" (13). Shifting from health to care requires an ethical disposition that recognizes bodies as spaces for intra-actional mattering. We need an ethic of care, therefore, that is sensitive to that which threatens lively relationalities of becoming. We need an ethic of care that treats as sacred the fragile ecological flux we always already share with a host of human and nonhuman agents. We need an ethic of care that interrupts "the slow death that happens to targeted or neglected populations over time and space" (Butler 2006, 169). The ongoing national disaster in Flint, Michigan, demonstrates that a body's well-being is not a thing an individual does or does not have.

Assumptions about bodies as individualistic entities with finite boundaries often warrant narratives of human choice and empowerment. Such narratives are especially prominent in discourse surrounding the promise of genetic or precision medicine. But bodies are "porous and not discretely bounded" (J. Brown 2015, 326). Care conducts well-being relationally. Feminist scholars in rhetorical theory and technical communication are uniquely positioned to challenge healthist discourses that are informed by myths of individualism. Atkinson et al. (2015) leverage the following indictment of the medical humanities, in particular: "While the medical humanities has done a lot to challenge dominant medical perspectives, it seldom if ever ventures beyond a neoliberal, humanist notion of the individual body-subject and associated conceptualizations of responsibility, rights, and risk management to really explore alternative 'collective' and 'relational' approaches to 'flourishing'" (77). Unlike the medical humanities, material feminists have always recognized the role of relationality—not only in biomedicine, but also in any debate about rights and equality. Ahmed (1996) makes the case that equality does not indicate sameness; rather, equality "constructs the subject as relational, as existing in connection with other subjects in a network of human relations" (75). To this network of human relations, I echo material feminists' addition of nonhuman and extrahuman actors.

Entanglements among humans, nonhumans, and extrahumans shape acts of diagnosis, prognosis, and treatment. Constant critical attention to how evincing disease is not a solely human enterprise but a matter of rhetorical attunement, in which evidences are coconstructed phenomena that emerge from material-discursive methods for making sense of the world, and in which care, not just health, is relational provides an ethical framework from which technical communicators, medical professionals, and other stakeholders might practice care. These three tenets might help care workers enact methods for tinkering within and among bodies that "cannot be definitively 'known' since" they are "not identical" with themselves "across time" (Gatens 1996, 57). After all, "the body does not have a 'truth' or a 'true' nature since it is a process and its meaning and capacities will vary according to its context. . . . These limits and capacities can only be revealed by the ongoing interactions of the body and its environment" (Gatens 1996, 57). Mol, Moser, and Pols (2010) provide numerous examples of what it looks like to practice care in a wide range of complex contexts—contexts that involve "living with the erratic" (10). Below I offer one additional possibility for what it looks like to live with the erratic, or to dwell with disease.

### DWELLING WITH DISEASE

We have at our disposal a plethora of constructs for understanding our interconnectedness, including Latour's collectives, Pickering's mangle, and Deleuze and Guattari's assemblage (to name only a few). What is needed now is the kind of transcorporeal ethic for which Alaimo (2008) advocates. Such an ethic rejects "disembodied values and ideals of bounded individuals" in exchange for "attention to situated, evolving practices that have far-reaching and often unforeseen consequences for multiple peoples, species, and ecologies" (Alaimo 2008, 253). Needed now is a kind of practical palimpsest—not a moral imperative or prescription—for how to be (a body) in the world in light of such an ethical disposition.

Disclosing, or shining a light on, that which *could be*, based on more than what *was*, requires radical presence. To dwell with disease is to be radically present and attuned to spatial and temporal contingencies of constantly changing phenomena. For Heidegger (1971), one cannot build or make unless one is capable first of dwelling. And for Ingold (2000), dwelling is embodied by "the forms people build" that, "whether in the imagination or on the ground, arise within the context of their involved activity, in the specific relational contexts of their practical engagement with their surroundings" (186). Heard (2013) describes dwelling more akin to a posture, habit, or identity (51) that requires attention not just to *techne* but also to physical, material contributors to that which he calls "tonality" and the ability to respond to others. Here, Heard's tonality echoes Davis's (2005) case for a "*non*-hermeneutical dimension of rhetoric that has nothing to do with meaning-making" (192). Davis argues: "Though I can neither appropriate nor fuse with you ... I must *respond* to you, orient myself toward you with seemingly boundless generosity" (200; italics in original). Being, making, and emplacement, therefore, are mutually constitutive acts. Dwelling, through the act not just of radical presence with but also radical response to disease and all its contributors, is one way of being attuned to and with a body in flux.

In many ways, we are always already dwelling with disease. In *Malignant: How Cancer Becomes Us*, Jain (2013) argues that those who have been diagnosed with cancer and are either in remission or have been cured "live in prognosis."[1] Here, cancer is more than a noun—cancer is "also a verb, an adjective, an invective, a shout-out, indeed, a grammar all its own" (Jain 2013, 223). While living in a constant state of prognosis, it's tempting to characterize cancer care as a kind of Sophoclean tragedy wherein medicine's practitioners merely play the role of chorus. Does living in a constant state of prognosis require relinquishing the future to little more than luck? Such was the case for Sophocles's *Antigone* who "lived on the razor's edge of luck" (Nussbaum 1989, 89). For the Greeks, luck wasn't necessarily the assertion that future events are random. Rather, *tuche* was what happened to a person not "through his or her own agency"; that is, *tuche* was "what just *happens* to him, as opposed to what he does or makes" (Nussbaum 1989, 3). *Tuche* might summarize the sense of powerlessness we feel in the face of a cancer diagnosis. In effect, *tuche* shifts the agential weight of extrahuman contributors in such a way that bodies are little more than passive stages on which disease does its thing.

As an ideological and practical counter to *tuche*, and given evidence-based medicine's "exuberant confidence in human power" (Nussbaum 1989, 89), contemporary medical practice relies on *technai*. *Technai*, at least in a classical rhetorical sense, is the deployment of human intelligence as a way to exert control over *tuche*. It makes human existence "safer, more predictable" and provides "a measure of control over contingency" (Nussbaum 1989, 91). *Technai* is "concerned with the management of need and with prediction and control concerning future contingencies" (Nussbaum 1989, 95). Within *technai*'s toolbox are such skills as systematicity, foresight, and experiential resources. A person guided by *technai* "possesses some sort of systematic grasp" or "some way of ordering the subject matter" (Nussbaum 1989, 95; see also Wickman [2012] for an extended discussion of *technai* in scientific inquiry). Systematicity, foresight, and experience are resources with which a person arrives to a situation, thereby making them "well prepared, removed from blind dependence on what happens" (Nussbaum 1989, 95). As we saw in each of this book's case studies, despite systematicity, foresight, and experience, indeterminacy persists. It is clear, therefore, that *technai* alone is insufficient for dwelling with disease.

Another way evidence-based medicine is characterized is through *episteme*. Dwelling with disease does not preclude *episteme* but instead recognizes *episteme*'s limitations. *Episteme* is typically translated as "knowledge, understanding; or science, body of knowledge" (Nussbaum 1989, 94) or, more specifically, a "deductive scientific understanding concerned with universals" (Nussbaum 1989, 299). Previous chapters demonstrated, however, that deductive, enthymematic reasoning does only so much to resolve medicine's indeterminacy. For all the ways deductive reasoning and scientific knowledge reveals, it simultaneously conceals. Is there a humane, habitable, and practical space between *tuche*, *technai*, and *episteme*? In this book's final pages, I explore such a question and posit several care-taking possibilities associated with *phronetic* medical practice as a method for dwelling with disease.

### Medical Practice as *Phronesis*

Among the constellation of rhetorical skills medical professionals deploy when attuning to bodies in flux, I have thus far described enthymematic reasoning, probabilistic *poesis*, *kairos*, and boundary work. To this list of rhetorical skills one might mobilize when attuning to bodies in flux, I now add *phronesis*. As Smith (2003) describes, *phronesis* is one of "the five expressions of care discussed in Book VI of the *Ethics*" and is a "mode that deals with the contingent and the possible" (83). Typically, *phronesis* (defined by Aristotle in the *Nicomachean Ethics* as "prudence") is set counter to another rhetorical construct, *metis*. In Greek mythology, Metis was once a resourceful and skillful female figure who, after literally being consumed by her husband, is reduced to no more than a disembodied voice in Zeus's head. Dolmage (2009) retells this myth and makes what I regard as a very important move to interrogate long-held assumptions about moral differences between *phronesis* and *metis*. That is, *metis*—typically defined as cunning intelligence, even trickery—is usually thought to be "bad *phronesis*" (Dolmage 2009, 11). Consequentially, "cunning intelligence must be made more systematic and epistemic to be acceptable" (Dolmage 2009, 11). Dolmage argues that by making *metis* "bad *phronesis*" we disembody if not dismiss such forms of intelligence (11). Herein lies the motivation to standardize and streamline ways of knowing: "bodily entailments must ... be made standard or tacit—not flexible and surprising" (11). Yet, Dolmage argues (and each of this book's case studies confirm) that bodily entailments are anything but static and predictable. Adding *phronesis* to the constellation of rhetorical skills necessary for contemporary medical practice does not, therefore, forfeit embodied knowing. Quite the opposite, in fact.

In classical rhetorical theory *phronesis* is often defined as practical wisdom—or a way of being in the world that is "resourceful at improvisation," sees "rules only as summaries and guides," and remains "flexible, ready for surprise," and "prepared to see" (Nussbaum 1989, 305). Smith (2003) argues that *phronesis* might be thought of as "a safeguard against a disposition (*hexis*) toward life that is unconcerned with everyday, practical needs in its pursuit of theoretical seeing ... *phronesis* is a way of being concerned with one's life (qua action) and with the lives of others—this is the purview of *praxis*" (88). It may be tempting to understand *phronesis* as a kind of flexible state of mind, or prudent judgment. When that temptation emerges, recall Dolmage's (2009) insistence that *phronesis* does not forfeit the agency of bodies. To such an insistence I add this: a material feminist practice of *phronesis* exceeds mind-body boundaries to include extrahuman environs. I argue that *phronesis* is a way of being (a body) in the world that is profoundly attuned to material *phainomena* and that to be attuned to such *phainomena* is "an openness to—a capacity to be affected-by-and-out-toward—aspects of a world" (Smith 2003, 83). Heard (2013) takes attunement into the realm of *phronesis* as I imagine it: "Attunement inclines us toward the synesthetic flood of tonality, the visual-aural-haptic conflation of sensory impressions that swells and cracks our capacity for meaning making" (59). Under the rubric of *phronesis*, then, care is not a disembodied morality or a right way of acting. It is radical dwelling in and through bodies, or a way of being inclined toward the flood of tonalities that bear up and make possible that which we come to know.

What might it look like to practice care as *phronesis*? What do such inclinations look like? Such radical dwelling with and response to? Consider the difficulty associated with caring for patients whose living conditions for one reason or another are perilously precarious. In such precarious care contexts, realities must be multiple. Lacking access to many of the technological and computational resources this book analyzes forces care workers in these scenarios, for instance, to see and use as scalpels and sutures technologies that are otherwise unintended for surgery. Such a care tactic is inherently improvisational. In her ethnography of an oncology ward in landlocked and impoverished Botswana, Livingston (2012) describes the challenge of improvising amid perilous material and socioeconomic contexts. Oncologists cared for patients affected by a sub-Saharan African cancer epidemic (which, to make matters worse, came on the heels of the HIV/AIDS epidemic). Broken machines, out-of-stock pharmaceuticals, and limited space necessitated improvisation. For Livingston, scientific methods for managing medical uncertainty are "an incomplete solution" (7). Dwelling with disease forces us—*all* of us—to step outside "pink ribbons, and invocations of cutting-edge research" that "sanitize cancer experiences" and to "find new ways to contemplate what it is to be seriously ill, extremely uncertain, and seeking relief" (Livingston 2012, 22). I concur with Livingston that this kind of care is "a highly contextualized pursuit" (6), a kind of "care" that is embedded within contexts of "debility and existential crisis"—or "a form of critical 'sociality based on incommensurate experience'" (Garcia 2010, 6). This kind of care invites us to reframe medical practice as *phronesis*, which "cannot be systematized like a *techne*" (Smith 2003, 89).

Practicing care as *phronesis* requires seeing what was and is as something more than an enthymematic premise for, or probabilistic predictor of, what will be. Attuning to "sociality based on incommensurate experience" (Garcia 2010, 6)—or what might be understood as the capacity to recognize multiplicity in practice (Mol 2002)—eschews attempts at controlling and cannibalizing the future (cf. Dunmire 2010). A material feminist understanding of *phronesis* requires that we "reimagine human corporeality, and materiality itself . . . as something that always bears the trace of history, social position, region, and the uneven distribution of risk" (Alaimo 2008, 261). What such a practice requires is an ethic of care that is sensitive and beholden to our transcorporeal condition. Matter, movement, and time intersect in precarious ways. Practicing care as *phronesis* is the act of attuning to such precarity (see Teston [2016] for an extended discussion of precarious rhetorics and contemporary medical practice).

Under the rubric of medical practice as *phronesis*, then, medical professionals practice being in the moment, or dwelling radically in such a way that they are concerned less with getting it right in the aggregate than getting it right locally. Medical professionals' radical attunement amid indeterminacy and contingency resists the guiding temptation to fear blame in a court of law. Medical professionals thereby accept statistical assessment and aggregated data as only "summaries and guides" (Nussbaum 1986, 305) and are permitted sensitivity to affect, emotion, and vulnerability. Medical professionals' actions and behaviors assume dependence on one another; they recognize that "we are all involved in affective and symmetrical relationships of care" (Winance 2010, 94)—to which I would add *a*symmetrical relationships of care. How best to "first, do no harm" than to attune to the effects of such asymmetrical relationships, recognizing that "independence is a fiction" (Winance 2010, 94)? Practicing care as *phronesis* means that care workers are rhetors who "take into consideration the worlds that people inhabit and the concerns that motivate those people" (Smith 2003, 86). What methods, then, do we use to evince the body when practicing care as *phronesis*?

Consider one example of what it might look like to evince a body under the rubric of medicine as *phronesis*, this time through the lens of disability. Imagine the seemingly quotidian yet complex act of fitting a patient who has a motor deficiency for a wheelchair. Winance (2010) gives an example of this process by describing the experiences of a patient named Mrs. Sabin. The wheelchair for which Mrs. Sabin had previously been fitted had, over time, become too small. Consequentially, Mrs. Sabin was quite uncomfortable and frequently suffered from back pain. Winance (2010) describes how Mrs. Sabin, her husband, and the wheelchair test center manager practice "trying a chair" by "experimenting, groping, and handling" (97); each actor "gradually shape[s] a person-in-a-wheelchair" and "tinker[s] around to make an arrangement" (101). In this practice of tinkering, "the actors act on the materiality of the person and the chair in an attempt to make them suit one another" (101). Here, not only is independence a fiction, but also "lack of fit reveals the ideological assumptions controlling the space" (Siebers 2008, 296). Such an act of backstage tinkering and acknowledging "lack of fit" is one example of what it might mean to evince the human body and all its disabilities. This is the *phronetic* practice of care. Smith (2003) says, "To engage a world 'phronetically' is, therefore, an attempt to understand its possibilities for relations and actions vis-à-vis the stable-mutable *phainomena* that comprise a world. It is an attending to the being-appearing of *phainomena*, that is, their movements of disclosure" (89). Doing care work within material-discursive mangles like these requires attunement to that which is local, material, affective, ideological, and socioeconomically conditioned.

Practicing *phronesis* does not seek to tune out extrahuman noise that might complicate statistical or standardizable generalizations. Rather, practicing *phronesis* brings forth a body as a collective—a collective that includes and necessitates attention to nonhuman noise. "To care is to tinker and to doctor. To care is to 'quibble,' to handle, to adjust, to experiment, to change tiny details in order to see if it works, to see if the person and the wheelchair can come to an arrangement and if they might get along with one another. … Here, care bespeaks a sensitivity shared and distributed among the actors. The object of care is not one single person but a collective" (Winance 2010, 102). *Phronetic* tinkering requires localized attunements and an uncomfortable, vulnerable, affective state of dwelling with dis-ease in a way management, control, and precision eschew. As Heard argues (2013), "attunement postures us to respond to the other even as we recognize the incompleteness of our response" (61). Here, the world is more "disclosed" than "constituted," and that "disclosure does not entail uncovering" or "getting reality right" but, rather, "bringing it to light" (Hekman 2008, 111). Medical practice as *phronesis*, therefore, means care workers doctor, tinker, and adjust while examining (if not comparing) the consequences of certain material-discursive phenomena over others.

It may seem as though tinkering and doctoring are obvious and apt constructs for describing wheelchair fitting as *phronesis*. But what about cancer care? In what ways do oncologists posture themselves to respond, to care—even as they "recognize the incompleteness" of such a response (Heard 2013, 61)? How, in oncologic care, does one tinker so that cellular chaos and human being "can come to an arrangement" (Winance 2010, 102)?

It is, indeed, possible even amid cancer-care flux to practice medicine as *phronesis*. To date, oncological science has made great strides in tinkering molecularly in the biomedical backstage. Already in some breast cancers, for example, scientists have found ways of treating cancer by tinkering with cells and other biological actors so that a body relies on its own agential capacity to heal itself. One of many promising areas of cancer research is immunology, or the study of how a body reacts and intra-acts with other biological and nonbiological entities. Immunology requires radical acceptance of bodies as collectives with distributed cellular, extracellular, and environmental actors. Such an approach is markedly different from the one with which we are most familiar: destruction and obliteration of cancer cells through pharmaceutical poison. No doubt there are other examples of how oncologic care in particular provides a practical palimpsest for how to be (a body) in the world.

Tinkering, care, and dwelling amid the whole network of relations (not just that which can be attuned to molecularly or computationally) is to practice medicine as *phronesis*. *Phronesis* is a way of being in a world full of "complex ambivalence and shifting tensions" (Mol, Moser, and Pols 2010, 14). After all, "*what is* is the process of becoming itself" (Bohm 1981, 61), and "what it is to be human has more to do with being fragile than with mastering the world"

(Mol, Moser, and Pols 2010, 15). As researchers in technical communication, rhetorical studies, medical rhetoric, medical humanities, and/or science and technology studies, we, too have a duty to advance an ethic of care that situates medical practice as *phronesis*. To do this we need more studies that demonstrate how doctors and other care workers can and do dwell with disease and all its multiplicity. No doubt we have carved hosts of "well-worn path[s] of critique" (Alaimo and Hekman 2008, 4). Needed now are more empirical studies, reports, and rigorously researched narratives of how care workers can and do attune to whole networks of relations.

In the conclusion of *Cruel Optimism*, Berlant (2011) describes the book's cover image, a painting by Riva Lehrer titled *If Body*. In this painting, a dog (Zora)—blind in one eye—is shown wearing a cone around her neck. Lying next to her on the ground is a woman (Riva). Riva, crippled by spina bifida, is shown weeping, covering half of her face. Reflecting on the image of Zora and Riva together, Berlant (2011) says,

> Zora and Riva seem at peace with each other's bodily being, and seem to have given each other what they came for: companionship, reciprocity, care, protection. Bodies make each other a little more possible: but they can't do everything. My sight can't give you your sight, my performative blindness may not even be empathy, and my mix of ability and impairment doesn't impinge much on yours. What we do have together, in the middle of this thing, is a brush with solidarity, and that's real.... A fantasy from the middle of disrepair doesn't add up to repair. It adds up to a confidence that proceeds without denying fragility. (266)

Oh, that we could exchange our ongoing desire for repair with confident solidarity. Attuning to and dwelling with—despite narratives of individualism, personalized medicine, and so-called scientific and medical progress—is, in the face of our collective fragility, to proceed with confidence in our togetherness. An ethic of care that champions medical practice as *phronesis* frames biomedical progress not necessarily in terms of precision but, rather, in terms of human fragility.[2] An ethic of care inspired by *phronesis* makes meaningful that which may resist aggregation. *Phronesis* forces us to recognize the role of matter, movement, and time in bodies' lively relationalities of becoming. In the face of persistent fragility and flux—"a world full of complex ambivalence and shifting tensions" (Mol, Moser, and Pols 2010, 14)—*phronesis* is the practice of dwelling confidently only in our togetherness; it is a method that neither denies fragility nor relies on vapid proclamations about beating or defeating disease.

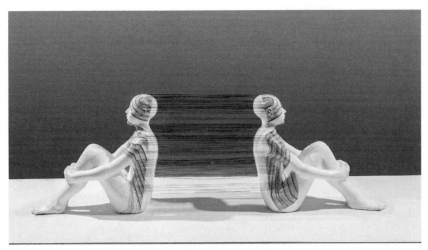

Figure 6.1 Tracey Sarsfield's *Reflected*

## Methodological Coda

It only makes sense that a book about methods for attuning to, being with, and dwelling among indeterminacy should close by commenting on methods for attuning to attunements. To illustrate such methods, consider sculptor Tracey Sarsfield's recent exhibition, *Reflected*.[3] In *Reflected*, Sarsfield explores the question, "when connecting with a fellow human being, what is it that we share?" In a way, Sarsfield examines—through resin, paint, fiberglass, and vinyl—multiple ontological spaces. Each of Sarsfield's sculptures show two human figures sitting across from and facing toward or away from one another, connected by black wires (fig. 6.1). Sarsfield's sculptures turn inside out the connections that were once invisible. This, too, is our trade: a kind of methodological cat's cradle challenge that, with every pass of the palm, turns mere strands or knots into structurally sound loops and layers.

As researchers, we must continue to tinker with methods for studying attunements, action, dwelling, and care. Methods for studying biomedical rhetorics ought to attune us to see care as an enterprise that both includes and transcends human doing (Rickert 2013, 83). Recall Latour's (2005) assertion that action is "a node, a knot, and a conglomerate of many surprising sets of agencies that have to be slowly disentangled" (44) and that we make a mistake when we "*ignore* the queerest, baroque, and most idiosyncratic terms offered by the actors, following *only* those that have currency in the rear-world of the social" (47; italics in original). As researchers of and practitioners in attuning to how others do things with things, our life's work hinges on a delicate sensitivity to otherwise invisible entanglements.

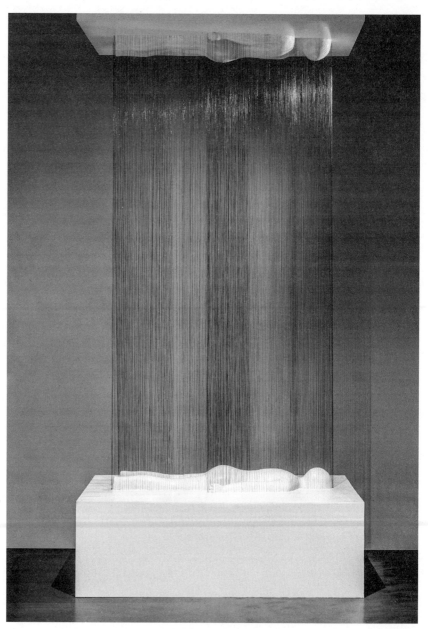

Figure 6.2 Tracey Sarsfield's *Rain*

One of Sarsfield's pieces in particular illustrates the kind of methodological moves for which I am advocating (see fig. 6.2). *Rain* displays two aligned figures with some distance between them, one facing downward, while the other faces upward. Connecting the two figures are hundreds of fishing lines. Each line's visible connection to both figures makes it difficult to discern (or decide) which direction the rain is actually moving, however. Is it falling from the top down, as one might expect? Or is it, counterintuitively, "falling" from the bottom up? Although most reviews want to read Sarsfield's exhibition as commentary about "the complexity of the self" (Haynes 2014, n.p.), one could also argue that *Rain* makes a case for movement, form, and being as a matter of connection. That which is connected is matter(ed).

And so, as we "follow power into places where current social theory seldom thinks to look for it—for example, in genes, climate models, research methods, cross examinations, accounting systems or the composition and practices of expert bodies" (Jasanoff 2004, 79–80)—we must remain mindful of the ways our methods for attuning to complexity shape human being. Those of us who study backstage, behind-the-scenes knots, lines that connect, and the queer spaces and places with which humans partner to make that which matters mean and that which means matter must find a way of dwelling with the flux and flow from both top down and bottom up.

# APPENDIX A. ODAC HEARINGS POST-AVASTIN, 2011–2013 (NOT INCLUDING PEDIATRIC HEARINGS)

| Hearing | Meeting Date | Issue | Proposed Indication | No. of Public Participants | Endpoints | Trials | Final Vote |
|---|---|---|---|---|---|---|---|
| 01 (a)[a] | 07/14/2011 (am) | BLA #125388 (ADCETRIS, a.k.a. Brentuximab Vedotin). Proposed by Seattle Genetics, Inc. | Treatment of relapsed or refractory Hodgkin lymphoma | 3 | Primary: ORR Secondary: CR Rate "What is the most appropriate primary endpoint in this trial (PFS or OS) to demonstrate clinical benefit?" (summary minutes of ODAC meeting, July 14, 2011, 5) | AETHERA: PFS is primary endpoint; powered to detect a PFS hazard ratio of 0.667, corresponding to a 6-month improvement in PFS; need an "adequate, validated quality of life instrument" if using PFS | 10+ (accelerated approval) |
| 02 (a)[a] | 07/14/2011 (pm) | BLA #125399 (ADCETRIS, a.k.a. Brentuximab Vedotin). Proposed by Seattle Genetics, Inc. | Treatment of relapsed or refractory systematic anaplastic large cell lymphoma | 2 | Primary: ORR Secondary: CR Rate "Some members discussed the appropriateness of PFS in these patients. One member mentioned a preference for OS as an endpoint, or PFS with a validated measure of patient-oriented outcomes. Other members felt that PFS is acceptable in these disease states, due to the limitations of measuring OS in this area" (summary minutes of ODAC meeting, July 14, 2011, 8) | Clinical trial SG035-0004 | 10+ (accelerated approval) |

| Hearing | Meeting Date | Issue | Proposed Indication | No. of Public Participants | Endpoints | Trials | Final Vote |
|---------|-------------|-------|---------------------|---------------------------|-----------|--------|-----------|
| 03[b] | 09/14/2011 (am) | NDA #021825 (Ferriprox, a.k.a. Deferiprone). Proposed by AcoPharma, Inc. represented by Cato Research Ltd. | Treatment of patients with transfusional iron overload when current chelation therapy is inadequate | 12 | Primary: 20% or greater decline per patient in serum ferritin after phase 1 therapy of up to 1 year. Secondary: 20% or greater improvement in liver iron concentration or cardiac T2* over the same time period | LA36–0310 (single, retrospective, uncontrolled, multi-institutional study) | Favorable risk/benefit profile? (10+, 2−) |
| 04 | 09/14/2011 (pm) | **DISCUSSION** | Re: patients with non-metastatic castration resistant prostate cancer who have rising serum level of PSA despite being on androgen deprivation therapy—potential trial designs and clinical endpoints | 2 | "Generally, members felt that three months of metastases-free survival was certainly insufficient, but that it was difficult to establish a clear demarcation for what duration of metastases prevention would be acceptable to prove clinical benefit" (summary minutes of ODAC meeting, September 14, 2011, 8). "Several members discussed problems with using time to symptomatic metastases as an endpoint. One member mentioned that this measure requires complicated and extensive follow-up and can be difficult to use in trials. An additional member discussed that the most common symptom in patients with metastases is fatigue rather than bony pain, making it very difficult to gauge the time to presentation of symptoms" (summary minutes of ODAC meeting, September 14, 2011, 8) | | NO VOTE |

| | Date | Application | Indication | | Endpoints | Discussion | Trials | Outcome |
|---|---|---|---|---|---|---|---|---|
| 05 (a) | 12/7/2011 (am) | NDA #202324 (INLYTA, a.k.a. Axitinib). Proposed by Pfizer Inc. | Treatment of patients with advanced renal cell carcinoma (RCC, kidney cancer) | 0 | Primary: PFS Secondary: OS | "Many members stated that overall survival and patient quality of life measures should be maintained as preferred outcomes in this patient population. Other members expressed some concern with measuring overall survival in these patients, with discussion of accrual difficulties, patient censoring, and heterogeneity of population cited as potential complications. One member discussed that measurement of overall survival may only be appropriate in high-risk patients, since other subsets may have life expectancies which make this measurement impractical. Several members indicated that, though overall survival and quality of life measures are the ideal outcomes to measure clinical impact, trials should also be designed with alternate outcomes to assist with validating these measures" (summary minutes of ODAC meeting, September 14, 2011, 8) | AXIS 1032 | Favorable risk/benefit profile? (13+) |
| 06[c] | 12/7/2011 (pm) | NDA #202799 (Peginesatide injection). Proposed by Affymax, Inc. | Treatment of anemia associated with chronic renal failure in adult patients on dialysis | 18 | Standard for efficacy=non-inferiority of hemoglobin levels | | Four randomized, active controlled studies (but other previous trials are brought to bear) | Risk/benefit favorable (15+, 1−) |

| Hearing | Meeting Date | Issue | Proposed Indication | No. of Public Participants | Endpoints | Trials | Final Vote |
|---|---|---|---|---|---|---|---|
| 07[d] | 2/8/2012 | sBLA #125329/28 (XGEVA, a.k.a. Denosumab). Proposed by Amgen Inc. | Treatment of men with castrate-resistant prostate cancer at high risk of developing bone metastases | 5 | Primary: Bone-metastases free survival Secondary: OS, patterns of metastases, development of symptomatic metastases | Placebo-controlled trial | Risk/benefit favorable (1+, 12−) |
| 08[e] | 2/9/2012 | sNDA 21790/010 (Dacogen, a.k.a. decitabine). Proposed by Eisai Inc. | Treatment of acute myelogenous leukemia in adults >65 years old, not candidates for induction chemotherapy | 0 | Study 016 PE: OS Study 017 PE: morphologic CR Secondary endpoints: demonstrating anti-leukemic activity | Study 016: phase 3, randomized, open-label, multicenter, multinational study Study 017 (supportive): phase 2, single-arm, open-label, multicenter study | Risk/benefit favorable (3+, 10−, 1 abstain) |
| 09[f] | 3/20/2012 (am) | sNDA 022465/S-010 (Votrient, a.k.a. pazopanib hydro-chloride). Proposed by Glaxo Wellcome Manufacturing Pte Ltd | Treatment of patients with advanced soft tissue sarcoma who have received chemotherapy | 1 | Primary: PFS Secondary: OS, ORR | Single, randomized study in patients with metastatic soft tissue sarcoma who received chemotherapy | Risk/benefit favorable (11+, 2−) |

| | Date | NDA/Drug | Indication | | Endpoint | Trial design | Risk/benefit |
|---|---|---|---|---|---|---|---|
| 10[g] | 3/20/2012 (pm) | NDA 022576 (Taltorvic, a.k.a. ridaforolimus). Proposed by Merck Sharp & Dohme Corp. | Treatment of adult and pediatric patients (13–17 years old, > 100 pounds) with metastatic soft tissue sarcoma or bone sarcoma as a maintenance therapy for patients who have completed at least 4 chemotherapy treatments without evidence of disease progression | 1 | Primary: PFS | Randomized trial in patients with metastatic soft tissue or bone sarcoma with SD following chemotherapy | Risk/benefit favorable (1+, 13–) |
| 11[h] | 3/21/2012 | NDA 202497 (Marqibo, a.k.a. vincristine sulfate liposomes injection). Proposed by Talon Therapeutics, Inc. | Treatment of adult patients with Philadelphia chromosome-negative acute lymphoblastic leukemia in second or greater relapse or whose disease has progressed following 2 or more treatment lines of anti-leukemia therapy | 0 | Single-arm phase 2 study: CR Phase 3 study: OS | Single-arm phase 2; randomized confirmatory global phase 3 open to enrollment | Risk/benefit favorable (7+, 4–, 2 abstain) |

| Hearing | Meeting Date | Issue | Proposed Indication | No. of Public Participants | Endpoints | Trials | Final Vote |
|---|---|---|---|---|---|---|---|
| 12[i] | 6/20/2012 (am) | NDA 203213. Proposed by Sanofi-aventis U.S. LLC. | Tx of prophylaxis of VTE in pts receiving chemo for locally advanced or mets pancreatic or lung cancer or for locally advanced or meta-static solid tumors with a VTE risk score of 3 or more | 1 | Primary: time to first occurrence of symptomatic DVT, nonfatal PE, or VTE-related death Secondary: OS at 1 year or at end of study | Single, randomized, placebo-controlled trial | Benefit/risk assessment: 1+, 14−, 1 abstain |
| 13[j] | 6/20/2012 (pm) | NDA 202714 (Kypro-lis, a.k.a. carfilzo-mib). Proposed by Onyx Pharma, Inc. | Treatment of patients with relapsed and refractory multiple myeloma who've received at least 2 prior lines of therapy | 10 | Primary: Overall response rate Secondary: clinical benefit response, duration of response (median), OS (median) | Single-arm, phase 2 trial; SUMMIT trial; APEX trial | Risk/benefit: 11+, 1 abstain |
| 14 (a) | 7/24/2012 | **DISCUSSION** Radiographic review in RCT using PFS as PE in nonhemato-logic malignancies | | 3 | "This approach assumes that INV-determined PFS could potentially be biased and, therefore, the role of IRC is to verify the INV assessments" (summary minutes of ODAC meeting, July 24, 2012, 4) | | NO VOTE Most mem-bers agreed that the presence of some sort of IRC review was critically important in recog-nizing and preventing bias. (5) |

| | | | | | | |
|---|---|---|---|---|---|---|
| 15 | 7/25/2012 | **Discussion/Vote** To what extent, if any, the presurgical ID of clear cell carcinoma of the kidney using an imaging test provides useful clinical information | 0 | "The test needs to have good performance characteristics (e.g., a sensitivity and specificity >80%)" (summary minutes of ODAC meeting, July 25, 2012) | | Yes: 16, Abstain: 1 |
| 16[k] | 5/2/2013 (am) | NDA 204408 (tivozanib capsules). Proposed by AVEO Pharma, Inc. | 9 | Treatment of advanced renal cell carcinoma | Primary: PFS Secondary: OS | Single, randomized trial | Risk/benefit (1+, 13−) |
| 17[l] | 5/2/2013 (pm) | NDA 201848 (drug/device combo, Melblez Kit). Proposed by Delcath Systems, Inc. | 1 | Treatment of patients with unresectable ocular melanoma that is metastasized to the liver | hPFS (hepatic PFS), overall PFS, OS | NCI phase 1 trial: open-label, single-center, multiple-ascending-dose | Risk/benefit (16−) |
| 18[m] | 5/3/2013 | **Discussion and Vote** | 0 | Safety and efficacy of currently approved LGF as potential treatments for radiation-induced myelosuppression associated with a radiological/nuclear incident | | All about whether the animal studies could be generalized to humans. | Clinical benefit in humans: (17+, 1−) |

| Hearing | Meeting Date | Issue | Proposed Indication | No. of Public Participants | Endpoints | Trials | Final Vote |
|---------|-------------|-------|--------------------|--------------------------|-----------|--------|-----------|
| 19 (a)[a] | 9/12/2013 | sBLA 125409/51 (Perjeta, a.k.a. pertuzumab). Proposed by Genentech, Inc. | Treatment in combo with trastuzumab and docetazel for neo-adjuvant treatment of patients with HER2+, locally advanced, inflammatory, or early stage breast cancer (tumor greater than 2 cm in diameter) as part of a complete early breast cancer regimen | 13 | Primary: pCR | NEOSPHERE (multi-center, randomized trial); 2 arms | Risk/benefit: 13+, 1 abstain |

Note: (a) = Avastin mentioned; BLA = biologics license application; ORR = objective response rate; CR = complete response; PFS = progression free survival; OS = overall survival; PSA = prostate specific antigen; NDA = new drug application; sBLA = supplemental biologics license application; sNDA = supplemental new drug application; SD = stable disease; DVT = deep vein thrombosis; VTE = venous thromboembolism; PE = pulmonary embolism; INV = investigator; IRC = independent radiological review committee; LGF = leukocyte growth factors; pCR = pathological complete response. Additional remarks from meeting minutes are flagged to the relevant hearing.

[a] Single-arm design and small size limit the benefit-risk analysis; time-to-event endpoints such as PFS or OS cannot be adequately interpreted in a single-arm trial; single-arm trial does not permit attribution of the adverse events; limited safety data.

[b] Retrospective nature of data; heterogeneity of the study population; lack of ongoing confirmatory trials; been marketed in the European Union since 1999 and other countries for similar indication.

[c] Study was unblinded.

[d] Several members felt that the difference in bone metastasis-free survival (BMFS) between the Denosumab (drug about which the deliberators debated; used to treat prostate cancer) and placebo arms of the trial was not large enough to establish clear clinical benefit. While there was some discussion of the appropriateness of BMFS as an established surrogate endpoint for clinical benefit, members generally agreed that it could be considered for this purpose because bone metastases can cause significant morbidity in patients with prostate cancer, but only if the magnitude was sufficient. One member stated that approximately one year difference in BMFS would be appropriate to establish clinical benefit. Several panel members concurred that the effect size demonstrated in the Denosumab trial was not of sufficiently large magnitude to establish clinical benefit, in the absence of a demonstrated effect on OS, PFS, or patient-reported outcomes (PROs) (summary minutes of ODAC meeting, February 8, 2012, 4).

<sup>e</sup>Members discussed whether the increased median overall survival seen in the trial could be considered a clinical benefit in light of the outcome not having reached statistical significance. Statistician panel members advised caution in interpreting outcomes that did not reach statistical significance and in assigning clinical importance to outcomes that were described by exploratory analyses. Generally, panel members agreed that statistical significance is not imperative for demonstration of clinical benefit, but that it is a major component in assessing the "big picture" of supportive evidence. Further, several members stated that it is critically important when considering a single trial that the results be consistent and robust (4). Some of these members stated that they felt that the analysis of median overall survival, though it did not meet statistical significance, was sufficient to encourage Decitabine's use in therapy. One member stated that it is difficult to be comfortable with a positive study result when one cannot be reasonably certain that the result is not based on random chance (summary minutes of ODAC meeting, February 9, 2012, 4).

<sup>f</sup>In regards to benefit, committee members discussed the value of a three-month improvement in PFS in this patient population. Members generally agreed that stabilizing these patients to be free of progression was valuable, but that the magnitude of the effect was marginal or modest at best. Some members discussed that other agents that are currently used off-label for treatment have had trouble achieving any real, measurable improvement in PFS in patients with advanced soft tissue sarcoma. In this context, some members expressed a sense that this three-month improvement in PFS represented a benefit to patients. Some members also cited the subset of patients who remained on treatment at one year as an indication of clinical benefit in the 14 percent of patients who comprised this subset. Members also discussed whether Pazopanib may improve quality of life or symptoms for these patients, but agreed that the data did not suggest this was the case (summary minutes of ODAC meeting, March 20, 2012, 4). Members who voted no expressed a feeling that the marginal effect demonstrated by the study did not conclusively represent a clinical benefit. One member stated that to prove benefit, a product should demonstrate impact on length or quality of life and that this trial did not do so conclusively (summary minutes of ODAC meeting, March 20, 2012, 4).

<sup>g</sup>In regards to the risk-benefit profile, several members expressed a perspective that maintenance therapies should meet a "higher bar" to demonstrate benefit, as this population would not otherwise be exposed to the toxicities of treatment. Many members stated that the magnitude of improvement in PFS was quite marginal and was unlikely to be clinically significant, despite having achieved statistical significance. Some members stated a feeling that the toxicities of the treatment would likely outweigh the benefit that was observed. Members discussed a desire for improvement in patient-reported outcomes, but concluded that the data did not support this (summary minutes of ODAC meeting, March 20, 2012, 7). Members who voted no consistently stated that the magnitude of PFS improvement in the trial was marginal and that this did not represent clinical benefit to patients when balanced against the existing toxicities. One of these members expressed discomfort with Ridaforolimus's place in therapy, stating that he would not feel comfortable treating a patient who had achieved stable disease with this drug. The member who voted yes expressed a desire to have more treatment options available and to preserve the availability of this product for patients (summary minutes of ODAC meeting, March 20, 2012, 8).

<sup>h</sup>Panel members expressed several different perspectives in regard to the risk-benefit profile of Marqibo. Several members discussed a lack of treatment options for the patient population that was studied and stated that these patients will often receive only supportive therapies. In this context, some members stated that the relatively small response rate would be greater than supportive care, where complete remission of the leukemia would not be seen. One member stated that the response rates seen with Marqibo may be similar to available combinations of active products but with fewer significant toxicities and with more convenient dosing and administration. Some members concurred that successfully bridging a patient to transplant did represent a real clinical benefit to those patients. Others on the panel expressed a feeling that the data from the trial did not conclusively demonstrate a clinical benefit to patients (summary minutes of ODAC meeting March 21, 2012, 4). Members who voted yes cited a feeling that the response rate in the trial was similar to the limited options that could otherwise be used in these patients but with less toxicity. Some of these members expressed that this, combined with a subset of patients being successfully bridged to transplant, represented a clinical benefit. Another member mentioned a possible benefit to patients in receiving a single agent rather than the multidrug regimen that would otherwise be used. One member stated that the yes vote was more an indictment of the lack of other options than enthusiasm about Marqibo (summary minutes of ODAC meeting, March 21, 2012, 4).

Members who voted no expressed doubt that the evidence was strong enough to suggest a reasonable likelihood of clinical benefit. One member cited skepticism of the pharmacology of the agent and its superiority to Vincristine, which is already available. Members who abstained from voting cited a lack of comfort with the quality of the data and a concern over questions that remained unaddressed (summary minutes of ODAC meeting, March 21, 2012, 5).

[i]A few members expressed a feeling that there likely is a target population that may benefit from the drug but that this population was not adequately established, or even suggested, by the single randomized trial (summary minutes of ODAC meeting, June 20, 2012, 4). In regards to benefit, some panel members expressed skepticism concerning the degree of clinical benefit described by the study results. Some of these members described a discomfort with the definition of DVT that was used in the study, stating that it likely included a large proportion of DVTs that were not clinically significant in light of the very serious disease state. One member stated that the negative quality-of-life impact of daily subcutaneous injections should be considered as well, because this will affect all patients receiving the prophylactic treatment (summary minutes of ODAC meeting, June 20, 2012, 5). Those who voted no expressed "doubt in the magnitude of benefit" (summary minutes of ODAC meeting, June 20, 2012, 5).

[j]Single-arm trial; refractory disease made risk acceptable.

[k]Members described difficulty with assessing data as a whole due to confounding aspects of the trial, including a unilateral crossover of patients to the sorafenib arm for post-study treatment. One committee member summarized the study results as demonstrating a questionable improvement in PFS with no demonstrable impact on quality of life and no demonstrated improvement in overall survival, with that impact possibly being negative (summary minutes of ODAC meeting, May 20, 2013, 4). A committee member expressed that any drug approval that is based on PFS should require a clear lack of ambiguity in the other aspects of the trial, which was not demonstrated in this case (summary minutes of ODAC meeting, May 20, 2013, 4). Concerns about generalizability to the United States since enrollment was low; limited exposure data in African American patients.

[l]"The treatment may be more toxic than the disease itself" (summary minutes of ODAC meeting, May 20, 2013, 8). The patient representative summarized this perspective by explaining a fear that approval of this product may offer "false hope" to patients with this disease, a statement that was supported by other members of the committee (summary minutes of ODAC meeting, May 20, 2013, 8).

[m]The animal study primary endpoint (survival) is clearly related to a desired benefit in humans. Committee members also believed that shortening the absolute neutrophil count recovery time is a useful supportive endpoint (summary minutes of ODAC meeting, May 3, 2013, 6). Some members recommended that additional beneficial information could be obtained to further refine the use of Filgrastim in the incident setting, as follows: (1) data from an animal model to establish clinical benefit based on the timing of leukocyte growth factor initiation following radiation, (2) data from a range of radiation doses, and (3) other investigations to further understanding of what would happen with the likely comorbidities (burns, trauma) in a nuclear incident scenario (summary minutes of ODAC meeting, May 3, 2013, 7).

[n]Many members touched on problems with pCR as an endpoint and uncertainty over whether this translates to long-term clinical benefit for patients (summary minutes of ODAC meeting, September 12, 2013, 5). They encouraged Genentech to voluntarily remove the indication if the confirmatory trial (named APHINITY) didn't confirm benefit.

# APPENDIX B. CSR OUTLINES

**Prostate Cancer**
1. Background
    a. Description of the condition
    b. Description of the intervention
    c. How the intervention might work
    d. Why it is important to do this review
2. Objectives
3. Methods
    a. Criteria for inclusion
        i. Types of studies
        ii. Types of participants
        iii. Types of interventions
        iv. Types of outcome measures
            1. Primary outcomes
            2. Secondary outcomes
    b. Search methods
        i. Electronic searches
        ii. Other resources
    c. Data collection and analysis
        i. Selection of studies
        ii. Data extraction and management
        iii. Assessment of risk of bias
        iv. Measures of treatment effect
        v. Dealing with missing data
        vi. Assessment of heterogeneity
        vii. Assessment of reporting biases
        viii. Data synthesis: random effects model
        ix. Subgroup analysis and investigation of heterogeneity
        x. Sensitivity analysis
4. Results
    a. Description of studies
        i. Results of the search
        ii. Included studies
        iii. Excluded studies
    b. Risk of bias in included studies (see Ilic et al. 2013, fig. 1)
        i. Allocation
        ii. Blinding
        iii. Incomplete outcome data

iv. Selective reporting

v. Other potential sources of bias

c. Effects of interventions

i. Prostate cancer-specific mortality

1. Results of meta-analysis (see Ilic et al. 2013, fig. 2)

2. Risk of bias-sensitivity analysis (see Ilic et al. 2013, fig. 3)

3. Subgroup analysis

ii. All-cause mortality

1. Results of meta-analysis (figure 4)

2. Risk of bias-sensitivity analysis

3. Subgroup analysis

iii. Diagnosis of prostate cancer (as determined by study)

1. Results of meta-analysis

2. Risk of bias-sensitivity analysis

3. Subgroup analysis

iv. Prostate tumor stage

1. Results of meta-analysis

2. Risk of bias-sensitivity analysis

v. Harms of screening

vi. Prostate grade distribution

vii. Quality of life and cost of screening

5. Discussion

a. Summary of main results

b. Overall completeness and applicability of evidence

c. Quality of the evidence

d. Potential biases in the review process

e. Agreements and disagreements with other studies or reviews

6. Authors' conclusions

a. Implications for practice

b. Implications for research

7. Acknowledgments

8. References

9. Characteristics of studies

a. Included (for each of five studies)

i. Methods

ii. Participants

iii. Interventions

iv. Outcomes

v. Notes

vi. Risk of bias

1. Bias

2. Authors' judgment

3. Support for judgment

b. Excluded studies characteristics
   i. Study/reason for exclusion
10. Data and analyses
   a. Screening versus control (for each analysis)
      i. Outcome/subgroup title
      ii. Number of studies
      iii. Number of participants
      iv. Statistical method
      v. Effect size
      vi. Risk ratios
      vii. Weight
      viii. Confidence intervals
11. Appendices
   a. Electronic database search strategy
12. What's new
13. History
14. Contributions of authors
15. Declarations of interest
16. Sources of support
   a. Internal
   b. External
17. Differences between protocol and review
18. Index terms
   a. Medical subject headings (MeSH)
   b. Medical subject headings check words

**Breast Cancer Screening**
1. Background
   a. Description of the problem (harms of unnecessary treatment of overdiagnosed tumors could reduce or outweigh potential benefits of screening)
   b. Description of the controversy
   c. Description of how meta-analyses of screening are deficient
2. Objectives
3. Methods
   a. Criteria for inclusion
      i. Types of studies
      ii. Types of participants
      iii. Types of interventions
      iv. Types of outcome measures
   b. Search methods
   c. Data collection and analysis
      i. Statistical methods

4. Results

    a. Description of studies

    b. Risk of bias in included studies (for each study)

        i. Population studied

        ii. Comparability of groups

        iii. Assignment of cause of death

        iv. Likelihood of selection bias

    c. Sources of data used for the meta-analyses

    d. Effects of interventions

        i. Deaths ascribed to breast cancer

        ii. Deaths ascribed to any cancer

        iii. All-cause mortality

        iv. Surgery

        v. Radiotherapy

        vi. Other adjuvant therapy

        vii. Harms

5. Discussion

    a. Breast cancer mortality

    b. Cancer mortality

    c. All-cause mortality

    d. Overdiagnosis and overtreatment

    e. False-positive diagnoses, psychological distress, and pain

    f. Other recent reviews of screening

    g. What were the absolute effects of screening in the trials?

    h. What is the effect of screening today?

6. Authors' conclusions

    a. Implications for practice

    b. Implications for research

7. Acknowledgments

8. References

9. Characteristics of studies

    a. Included (for each of five studies)

        i. Methods

        ii. Participants

        iii. Interventions

        iv. Outcomes

        v. Notes

        vi. Risk of bias

            1. Bias

            2. Authors' judgment

            3. Support for judgment

    b. Excluded studies characteristics

        i. Study/reason for exclusion

10. Data and analyses
    a. Screening versus control (for each analysis)
        i. Outcome/subgroup title
        ii. Number of studies
        iii. Number of participants
        iv. Statistical method
        v. Effect size
        vi. Risk ratios
        vii. Weight
        viii. Confidence intervals
11 What's new
12. History
13. Contributions of authors
14. Declarations of interest
15. Sources of support
    a. Internal
    b. External
16. Differences between protocol and review
17. Index terms
    a. MeSH
    b. MeSH check words

**Lung Cancer Screening**
1. Background
    a. Description of the condition
    b. Description of the intervention
    c. How the intervention might work
    d. Why it is important to do this review
2. Objectives
3. Methods
    a. Criteria for inclusion
        i. Types of studies
        ii. Types of participants
        iii. Types of interventions
        iv. Types of outcome measures
    b. Search methods
        i. Electronic searches
        ii. Other resources
    c. Data collection and analysis
        i. Selection of studies
        ii. Risk of bias
4. Results
    a. Description of studies

b. Risk of bias in included studies (see Manser et al. 2013, figs. 1 and 2)

    i. Randomization

    ii. Blinding of outcome assessment

    iii. Description of withdrawals and dropouts

    iv. Statistical analysis

    v. Agreement between authors on methodological quality (using kappas)

c. Effects of interventions

    i. Lung cancer mortality

        1. Mort intense chest X-ray screening compared with less intense chest X-ray screening

        2. Annual chest X-ray screening versus usual care (no screening)

        3. Annual low-dose CT screening versus chest X-ray screening

    ii. All-cause mortality

        1. More intense versus less intense

        2. Annual chest X-ray versus no screening

        3. Annual low-dose CT screening versus annual chest X-ray screening

    iii. Compliance with screening and contamination in the control group

    iv. Number of cases of lung cancer detected

    v. Survival

    vi. Stage distribution

    vii. Resection rates

    viii. Postoperative deaths and harm associated with screening

    ix. Costs

    x. Quality of Life

    xi. Test performance

    xii. Smoking behavior

    xiii. Consumer perspectives

5. Discussion

6. Authors' conclusions

    a. Implications for practice

    b. Implications for research

7. Acknowledgments

8. References

9. Characteristics of studies

    a. Included (for each of five studies)

        i. Methods

        ii. Participants

        iii. Interventions

        iv. Outcomes

        v. Notes

        vi. Risk of bias

1. Bias
2. Authors' judgment
3. Support for judgment
   b. Excluded studies characteristics
      i. Study/reason for exclusion
10. Data and analyses
    a. Screening versus control (for each analysis)
       i. Outcome/subgroup title
       ii. Number of studies
       iii. Number of participants
       iv. Statistical method
       v. Effect size
       vi. Risk ratios
       vii. Weight
       viii. Confidence intervals
11. Appendices
    a. Electronic database search strategies for each version of review
12. What's new
13. History
14. Contributions of authors
15. Declarations of interest
16. Index terms
    a. MeSH
    b. MeSH check words

# APPENDIX C. GENETIC TESTING METHODS AND TECHNIQUES, 1950–1990

| Date | Method | Technique |
|------|--------|-----------|
| 1950 | Edman degradation | Reagents were used to sequence amino acids of proteins. This was a manual process in which phenylisothicyanate (PITC) was used in conjunction with weak acids to cleave the protein in order, amino acid by amino acid. Scientists then used chromatograph to determine identity. |
| 1958 | Automated chronography | Scientists used Armour crystalline RNA (from Armour meat-packing company) to sequence RNA. They used an ion exchange chromatograph and broke each peptide into fragments, cleaved them with reagents, and ran samples in an ion exchange chromatograph. |
| 1975 | Plus and minus (Sanger) | A primer was extended by a polymerase to generate a population of newly synthesized deoxyribonucleotides of assorted lengths; the unused deoxyribonucleotides were removed, and polymerization continued in four pairs of plus and minus reaction mixtures. |
| 1976 | Maxam and Gilbert Method | Scientists used base-specific chemicals to cleave. They used radioactive markers, randomly cleaved each strand with one of four base-specific chemicals. |
| 1977 | Sanger dideoxy sequencing | Scientists took sample DNA, added primer and DNA polymerase to each tube containing a specific dideoxynucleotide, ran contents of each tube through separate lanes of gel electrophoresis, and determined the position of the base. The lanes of the gel acted as stand-ins for a strand of DNA. |
| 1980s | Hood and Hunkapiller | Scientists used four different fluorescent dyes to label each nucleotide, allowing electrophoresis to be run in a single lane (Lee et al. 2013, 92). Detection with laser/camera unit was highly automated since the bright colors could be detected with precision. |
| 1990s | Lander's technique | Scientists developed bead-based preparations to capture DNA. They cracked cells open, put in beads, and the beads binded to DNA. |

# NOTES

1. Interestingly, prior to settling on "evidence-based medicine" as a name, Guyatt's proposal for elevating critical appraisals above expert opinion was originally called "scientific medicine." According to Smith and Rennie (2014), faculty at McMaster "reacted against this name with rage, arguing that basic scientists did scientific medicine."

2. Here and throughout, I use "complex" not simply to indicate that something is complicated but, rather, to describe a thing that, according to Rickert (2013), "cannot be adequately analyzed through or predicted from the component elements but rather enters a new state of order or equilibrium that transcends the initial state" (100). The complexity of the human body or cancer, specifically, is a part of the contingent, indeterminate flux with which medical professionals and patients grapple.

3. I understand that different hospitals have varying ways of managing tumor board conferences. At a much larger teaching hospital, e.g., one tumor board conference meeting was devoted strictly to breast cancer. Here, patients were referred to by number, charts were used to guide discussion, and deliberators spent no more than five minutes per patient determining the best course of action. These kinds of tumor board meetings are quite different from the ones that the local community hospital holds. The latter inspires this book.

4. See Teston (2012b).

5. Regarding the deliberative process, see Teston (2012a).

6. See also Barton (2004).

7. Augury is the practice of interpreting the will of the gods by studying birds' flight patterns.

8. I am indebted to medical historian Susan Lawrence for this reference.

9. Indeed, Sara Ahmed reiterated this three times to her audience of which I was a part at a recent lecture as she read passages from Descartes and reminded us of the obstinate arm and the disciplining switch from the Grimm Brothers' "Willful Child."

10. For a focus on humans, see Lynda Walsh's (2013) *Scientists as Prophets*.

11. Latour (1987) describes these alliances as networks. "The word network indicates that resources are concentrated in a few places—the knots and the nodes—which are connected with one another—the links and the mesh: these connections transform the scattered resources into a net that may seem to extend everywhere" (180).

## CHAPTER TWO

1. The estimate of how many cells are in a human body fluctuates drastically depending on the metric (e.g., volume vs. weight) used for measurement (see chap. 3 for an analysis of how metrics and other measures for assessment affect findings).

2. In *Vibrant Matter*, Bennett (2010) highlights what she says is "typically cast in the shadow: the material agency or effectivity of nonhuman or not-quite-human things" (ix).

3. Haghighian (2006) cautions against declaring these processes "invisible," since such a characterization implies a "voilà approach" that "creates a misconception, a blindness in front of the object—blindness to the complex relationship between invisibility and visualization and to the various realities of the object under observation" (67).

4. Borrowing from Farkas and Haas, I use slashes rather than bullets to delineate codes or data points.

5. Cancer staging is an evaluative assessment that ultimately determines how aggressively a patient should be treated.

6. Readers might be familiar with similar claims that are grounds on which Heisenberg's uncertainty principle and the observation effect are made.

7. Although this chapter is careful not to collapse the cellular body with particle physics, Knorr Cetina (2009) describes how the laboratory reconfigures both the very organic objects that scientists examine and scientists, themselves. She explores how "scientists and other experts" are "enfolded in construction machineries" (11) and argues that "we need to conceive of laboratories as processes through which reconfigurations are negotiated, implemented, superseded, and replaced" (45). Technologies and methods for seeing (and knowing) are not impotent or passive tools used by a human agent. Instead, medical professionals and scientists partner with "obscure work, instruments, and disciplined bodies" (Callon, Lascoumes, and Barthe 2009, 57) when attuning visually to phenomena—phenomena whose emplacement and material makeup evolve persistently in spite of cutting-edge technological scopes and scans. Such assertions require rethinking long-standing beliefs about subject-object relationships.

8. Happe (2013) leverages this critique quite persuasively by making the case that "environmental genomics research assumes that pollution is an inevitable feature of modern life, a naturalized feature that has no history, no politics, and no thinkable solutions—indeed, it ceases to be thought of as pollution at all. Instead, inherited genetic mutations are the polluting agents, a conceptual displacement that is part and parcel of a neoliberal logic that valorizes personalized, market-driven medical and public health interventions" (140).

9. As a first step in shedding what she refers to as "anthropocentric moorings," Barad (2007) argues that we must cease theorizing objects as being independent, or having "inherent boundaries and properties" (333). Barad proposes that we imagine these once-bounded objects as "phenomena." She asserts that "phenomena do not merely mark the epistemological inseparability of 'observer' and 'observed'; rather, *phenomena are the ontological inseparability of intra-acting 'agencies.'* That is, *phenomena are ontological entanglements*" (333; italics in the original). For Barad, "particular material articulations of the world become meaningful" as a result of "specific agential intra-actions" (333). Researchers in technical commu-

nication, medical humanities, and rhetorical theory can understand such agential intra-actions through analyses of methods for resolving biomedical indeterminacy, although these observations as well are but partial perspectives.

10. And dwelling requires remembering the political, cultural, and historical background of cellular materiality and ways in which, among other things, "race, gender, and (dis)ability profoundly shape the very nature of . . . scientific speculation" (J. Brown 2015, 328).

11. In *One Renegade Cell*, Weinberg (2013) notes that "most human tumors comprise a billion or more cells before we become aware of them" (quoted in Belling 2010, 229).

12. Landecker (2007) invites readers to consider the way cells are a kind of proxy "for the patients from which they have been extracted" (2).

CHAPTER THREE

1. Avastin is what is known as an angiogenesis inhibitor. That means that rather than act directly on a tumor by shrinking it or limiting its growth, it inhibits the formation of new blood vessels that would bring vital nutrients to a growing cancer. As such, it has been widely hailed as an important weapon in the fight against various metastatic cancers. Originally approved by the FDA for the treatment of colorectal cancer in 2004, Avastin was the first angiogenesis inhibitor developed and available on the market. Given its novelty and purported efficacy, it has been a widely popular in the treatment of a variety of cancers, including colorectal, ovarian, and breast.

   In 2008, the FDA approved Avastin specifically for the treatment of breast cancer under the accelerated approval process. The typical FDA drug approval process frequently requires many years of study. Under the normal process, proposed drugs must endure four phases of clinical trials designed to assess their safety, efficacy, and proper dosage. Recognizing that the rigorous and lengthy nature of this process may delay approval beyond the lifespan of many current patients with terminal disorders, in 1992, the FDA launched an accelerated approval process. The drawback of this process is that approval is provisional. Drug makers must continue to perform the standard four-phase trial process and eventually secure full approval. In the case of Avastin, however, these follow-up trials, called confirmatory trials, failed to convince the FDA to issue full approval, and they subsequently revoked the breast cancer indication in 2010. This caused even further outcry and a special appeal hearing was convened on June 28 and 29, 2011. This special meeting included testimony form the manufacturer and cancer experts as well as a half day of nonvoting members of multiple publics, including patients, survivors, and family members. These stakeholders' testimonies failed to be taken up in the expert panel's final deliberative process, and the revocation of the breast cancer indication for Avastin was upheld and confirmed on November 18, 2011.

2. This chapter's analyses are new. They do, however, build on events described in two previous publications (Teston and Graham 2012; Teston et al. 2014).

3. The video and written transcripts of the Avastin Hearing are publicly available at http://www.fda.gov/newsevents/meetingsconferencesworkshops/ucm255874 .htm. Results of this hearing were strictly advisory. The ultimate decision authority was located with a single individual, the commissioner of the FDA, Margaret Hamburg. Commissioner Hamburg issued her final decision, which followed the Oncologic Drugs Advisory Committee's recommendation, on November 18, 2011.

4. National Cancer Institute, "NCI Dictionary of Cancer Terms," http://www.cancer .gov/publications/dictionaries/cancer-terms?cdrid=44070.

5. This doesn't mean Avastin is missing from the market. Avastin use is still approved as a treatment option for other cancers. And oncologists may choose to continue using Avastin in the case of end-stage breast cancer; the patient would have to foot the bill for the cost since insurance companies will not reimburse providers who use a medication for an indication unapproved by the FDA.

6. I should clarify that I aim not to adopt an accusatory stance toward bureaucratic organizations such as the FDA that invoke impersonal methods of statistical analysis when assessing the meaningfulness of certain kinds of evidence. Surely, enough of these kinds of whistle-blowing critiques based on ex cathedra rhetorical analyses exist (including my own earlier publications on the Avastin pharmaceutical hearing).

7. Shifting the definition of rhetoric to include not only the symbolic art of persuasion but also a method for becoming evidentially attuned rescues material practices such as the statistical construction of clinically meaningful endpoints from "anthropocentric moorings" (Barad 2007, 334). That is, we are no longer limited to attributing deliberative disagreements between experts and nonexperts to a drug company's concern about their bottom line or a policy wonk's callousness. Indeed, bottom lines and insensitivity to patient reports may very well exist. But taking to be true both Rickert's and Barad's arguments about the meaningfulness of material performances of the world, there are other contributors to the disagreement present during pharmaceutical assessments.

8. Welhausen and Burnett (2016) have an excellent chapter about smallpox, risk, and the history of statistical graphics wherein they trace how visual displays of quantitative information organize, shape, and design information in such a way that decisions might be made. In particular, they analyze visual displays of smallpox risk through the rubric of correlation, location, and value.

9. I am indebted to Candice Lanius for her feedback on an early draft of this chapter. Her expertise in statistics and rhetoric was quite valuable.

10. While risk analyses, cost benefit analyses, and quality-of-life analyses certainly exist, there is not yet a well-controlled assessment mechanism by which these data might be incorporated meaningfully into pharmaceutical deliberations as evidence.

11. Transcripts of the various ODAC meetings can be found by clicking on the meeting year in the list at left at http://www.fda.gov/AdvisoryCommittees/Committees MeetingMaterials/Drugs/OncologicDrugsAdvisoryCommittee/default.htm.

12. Engeström (1993) defines activity theory not as a "specific theory of a particular domain, offering ready-made techniques and procedures." Rather, he sees it as a "general, cross-disciplinary approach, offering conceptual tools and methodological principles, which have to be concretized according to the specific nature of the object under scrutiny" (97).

13. Bayesian statistics—a different statistical assessment method that the FDA uses only when assessing the efficacy and safety of medical devices—can actually provide probabilities about future events. The branch of statistics I discuss in this chapter is frequentist statistics.

14. Similarly, Rotman (2000) argues that "mathematics involves creation of imaginary worlds that are intimately connected to, brought into being by, notated by, and controlled through the agency of specialized signs" (ix) and that "mathematical assertion is a prediction" (16).

15. In *Acting in an Uncertain World*, Callon, Lascoumes, and Barthe (2009) propose that scientific researchers are part of a larger "research collective" wherein intelligence is distributed. Specifically, they argue, "what human beings can say and write, what they can assert and object to, cannot be dissociated from the obscure work of the instruments and disciplined bodies that cooperate and participate in their own right in the elaboration of knowledge" (57). Note here Callon, Lascoumes, and Barthe's emphasis on how the work of "instruments and disciplined bodies" cooperate and participate *in their own right*. The authors are careful to not overdetermine the notion of intelligence—especially *human* intelligence—within this research collective: "Reference to the notion of distributed intelligence enables one to distribute the skills usually attributed to researchers across a multiplicity of other actors, and non-human actors in particular. But it runs the risk of a possible misinterpretation induced by the word 'intelligence.' The reader will have understood that it is not only intellectual, and even less cerebral capabilities that are distributed, but also and above all embodied forms of know-how, knacks, knowledge crystalized in various materials, and craft skills" (2009, 58).

16. Some readers may wonder why I refrained from evaluations of accusations about the FDA's moral failing in their perceived unwillingness to incorporate breast cancer survivors' testimony into their deliberations. Let me attend to this problem by stating plainly that I am not willing to concede that the conundrum in which the FDA found itself was the result of nothing more than the rumored decades-long tiff between Genentech (the pharmaceutical company that developed Avastin) and the FDA, or their perceived insensitivity to women's testimony. Certainly, unveiling power dynamics and dominant discourses are important and worthy intellectual pursuits. However, I propose that methods of evidential attunement ultimately shape what it is we can or cannot see—*not necessarily what we will or will not see.*

Managing medical uncertainty hinges largely on our capacity (or lack thereof) to extract a meaningful signal from a sea of noise. Inferential statistics got its big break, as Bram (2014) explains, with Fisher's agricultural experiments in the 1920s. In an effort to determine which fertilizers would yield greater crops, Fisher

(1921) devised a method for assessing the quality of particular inferences. Even when his dependent and independent variables stood still (i.e., while the fertilizer a farmer used would affect how much corn grew, corn growth could never influence fertilizer), methods for bringing out of concealment into unconcealment had to be devised. In other words, there are some things you just cannot eyeball. Like Fisher, medical statisticians are constantly honing methods with greater sensitivity for extracting signal from noise. These methods are part of whence our problem comes.

Flattening rhetorical events such as pharmaceutical hearings into discursive battlefields limits rhetoric to little more than a symbolic art. So in addition to identifying how methods of evidential attunement—specifically, inferential statistics— "bring the world into rhetorical performance" (Rickert 2013, xviii), this chapter also characterizes rhetoric as both epistemological and ontological; rhetoric does double duty by not only persuading interlocutors of the value of a certain truth or reality but also attuning them to see such truths or realities in the laboratory, in the first place.

## CHAPTER FOUR

1. One communication studies scholar, Everett Rogers, developed a theoretical framework, "diffusion of innovations," for investigating this gap. According to Rogers (1962), there are five stages to adopting new innovations: knowledge, persuasion, decision, implementation, and confirmation.

2. I am indebted to William Hart-Davidson and Margaret Holmes-Rovner, both of whom introduced me to the important role CSRs play in medical practice. In the beginning stages of a collaborative, exploratory study of how medical professionals manage the arduous task of synthesizing evidences, I learned how evidences from various clinical trials and across multiple sources were synthesized so that medical professionals could arrive at evidence-based medical recommendations about the efficacy of interventions.

3. In this chapter, as opposed to "uncertainty," I will deploy "indeterminacy" as an investigative construct. The use of "indeterminacy" is motivated by Barad's (2007) discussion of Bohr's two-slit experiment. "For Bohr, there's nothing mysterious about wave-particle complementarity; it's simply a matter of the material specificity of the experimental arrangement that gives meaning to certain classical variables to the exclusion of others, enacts a specific cut between the object and the agencies of observation, and produces a determinate value of the corresponding property" (Barad 2007, 268; italics in original). Cancer-care flux is resolved by rhetorically establishing "determinate values." For both Bohr and Barad, determinate values are not just discursive; they are also material cuts.

4. See app. B for outlines of each CSR.

5. See chap. 3 for a detailed analysis of statistical methods for making clinical trial data matter and mean.

6. Cicero, *De Inventione*, DOI: 10.4159/DLCL.marcus_tullius_cicero-de_inventione.1949; Quintilian, *Institutio Oratoria*, trans. H. E. Butler (London: William Heinemann, 1921).

CHAPTER FIVE

1. According to the National Cancer Institute, BRCA1 and BRCA2 mutations combined account for 5–10 percent of all breast cancers and about 15 percent of ovarian cancers. Detecting a variation in one of these two genes does not necessarily mean that someone will develop breast or ovarian cancer. While rare, these variations are not necessarily mutations. If a BRCA1 mutation is found, it is estimated that there is a risk of up to 80 percent over the course of a person's lifetime for being diagnosed with breast cancer and a 50 percent chance of being diagnosed with ovarian cancer. Being able to detect genetic variations in either of these two (or more) genes can be powerful predictors of a woman's health and her response to particular oncologic interventions.

2. Happe (2013) might refer to this as the "privatization of risk" (140).

3. A single gram of DNA is approximately 5.5 petabits of data, or approximately 700 terabytes.

4. The policy states: The term "device"—except when used in paragraph (n) of this section and in sections 301(i), 403(f), 502(c), and 602(c)—means an instrument, apparatus, implement, machine, contrivance, implant, in vitro reagent, or other similar or related article, including any component, part, or accessory, which is— (1) recognized in the official National Formulary, or the U.S. Pharmacopeia, or any supplement to them, (2) intended for use in the diagnosis of disease or other conditions, or in the cure, mitigation, treatment, or prevention of disease, in man or other animals, or (3) intended to affect the structure or any function of the body of man or other animals, and which does not achieve its primary intended purposes through chemical action within or on the body of man or other animals and which is not dependent upon being metabolized for the achievement of its primary intended purposes.

5. "Receiving 'Variant Not Determined' or 'Result Not Determined' in a Report," 23andMe.com, https://customercare.23andme.com/hc/en-us/articles/212196558 -Receiving-Variant-not-determined-or-Result-not-determined-in-a-report.

6. See https://getcolor.com/blog/2015/08/diversity-is-in-our-dna.

7. In 2013, Myriad Genetics—Color Genomics' biopower predecessor—appealed to the Supreme Court for legislation that would allow them to renew their patent on BRCA1 and BRCA2. Myriad Genetics is a genetic sequencing company that has forged unprecedented ground by honing analyses that focus specifically on genes whose variations (or what the popular press falsely refers to as "mutations") are associated with increased risk for breast and ovarian cancer. Two of those genes are BRCA1 and BRCA2. Were they granted the rights once more to patent these genes, they could monopolize this particular corner of the genetic testing market. Myriad

stood to profit a good deal given their association with Jolie's decision and resultant *New York Times* op-ed. The Supreme Court rejected Myriad's patent renewal. Since then, venture capitalists helped fund one of Myriad's main competitors: a startup genetic testing corporation called Color Genomics. Unlike Myriad, Color Genomics sells genetic testing kits directly to the consumer. These tests, based on their genetic sequencing techniques, render evidences from very large data sets that can then be used to support probabilistic claims about a consumer's risk of developing (or at least being diagnosed with) breast and ovarian cancer.

8. See app. C for a history of genetic testing methods and techniques, 1950–90.

9. What might happen if we mapped the inescapable history of the eugenics movement on top of these relationships? How might that complicate these concepts and their intra-actions? The door is wide open for these kinds of inquiries.

10. Like Clarke et al. (2010), I do not see technology as deterministic. Rather, I make the assumption, in this chapter, that "sciences and technologies are made by people and things working together" (55).

11. Claims about the actual heritability of a particular disease, such as breast cancer, as can be derived (not determined) from SNP genotyping, are not as reliable as whole genome or exome sequencing. Whereas in exome or whole genome sequencing scientists can detect variations in single nucleotides (called SNVs), with DNA profiling using SNPs, scientists are only able to detect variations that occur in at least 1 percent of the population. This may seem perfectly acceptable, except for the fact that this population is a fraction of a fraction of an actual population.

12. In almost every nucleus of every human cell there is a full copy of one's genetic makeup. This is called a genome. A genome contains twenty-three chromosomes. In each chromosome there are 48–250 million nucelobases, each of which are identified as one of the following: adenine, cytosine, guanine, thymine. Variations in the order of those nucelobases are what result in human differences. When those differences are visible, it's referred to as a phenotype. The underlying genetic expressions that make those differences visible (and in most cases *invisible*) are, in contrast, referred to as a genotype.

13. Day (2014) argues that, "the 'gathering up' or sublimation of qualitative being, work, affects, and relationships into quantitative, algorithmic, devices often proves insufficient for addressing the ontological values of the former, whether this concerns friendship, understanding, or any other relationship that 'takes time'" (128; italics in original).

14. Exome sequencing relies on markedly different technologies and methods than those of whole genome sequencing. As the name suggests, whole genome sequencing involves sequencing the whole genome (not just the exome). Whole genome sequencing is a timely and costly endeavor. At this time, available direct-to-consumer genetic tests for sequencing the whole genome are less popular and much more expensive (approximately $5,000). By sequencing whole genomes and then comparing the results of, say, your genome sequence with your mother's and grandmother's, scientists can establish the frequency of certain mutations. Scientists

estimate that every generation involves the mutation of approximately seventy genes. In the exome, scientists estimate there are only 0.35 mutations that change protein sequences between parents and their children. Cancerous cells, however, mutate much more frequently than noncancerous cells.

15. This is important because increasingly when news media report on genetic discoveries, especially as they relate to disease, they (erroneously) refer to benign genetic variations as a mutation. Genetic variation is not an aberrant phenomenon.

16. Consider W. Brown's (2015) admonition: "Neoliberalization is more termitelike than lionlike ... its mode of reason boring in capillary fashion into the trunks and branches of workplaces, schools, public agencies, social and political discourse, and above all, the subject" (35–36).

17. In studying how texts are put together to achieve their effects, rhetoricians often appear to imply premeditated calculation on the author's part. But as Ceccarelli (2001) points out, "Just as an organism might adopt a successful evolutionary strategy without being consciously aware of it, so too might an author adopt a successful rhetorical strategy without being consciously aware of it" (5).

18. As Bateson (1994) says: "Trusted habits of attention and perception may be acting as blinders" (8).

19. For Beck (1999), the politics of risk is "a form of organized irresponsibility." Mindful of this, Scott (2006) makes the case that managing risk is a rhetorical process that "usually involves building networks of heterogeneous risk objects" (121). And indeed, direct-to-consumer genetic testing corporations advertise risk management through a network of mostly invisible heterogeneous risk objects—objects this chapter explores.

20. Herein lies the importance of technical communicators whose backgrounds include rhetorical theory.

## CHAPTER SIX

1. For a discussion on rhetorics of hope in prognosis, see Barton and Marback (2008).

2. Regarding fragility, Sara Ahmed (2010) said it best in a lecture she gave at Kent University. I struggle to paraphrase her words because I'm still processing their implications. She suggests that "perhaps from fragility we can think of other ways of building feminist shelters. We might think of fragility not so much as the potential to lose something, fragility as loss, *but as a quality of relations we acquire, or a quality of what is we build.* A fragile shelter has looser walls, made out of lighter materials; see how they move. A movement is what is built to survive what has been built. When we loosen the requirements to be in a world, we create room for others to be."

3. The exhibition can be found on her website, http://www.traceysarsfield.com/.

# REFERENCES

Ahmed, S. 1996. "Beyond Humanism and Postmodernism: Theorizing a Feminist Practice." *Hypatia* 11 (2): 71–93.

———. 2015. "Self-Care as Warfare: Fragility, Militancy, and Audre Lorde's Legacies." Lecture, Kent University, December 10. https://player.kent.ac.uk/Panopto/Pages /Viewer.aspx?id=9232575d-61dc-48de-8c4e-5e07b6a3a9d5.

Alaimo, S. 2008. "Trans-corporeal Feminisms and the Ethical Space of Nature." In *Material Feminisms*, edited by S. Alaimo and S. Hekman, 237–64. Bloomington: Indiana University Press.

Alaimo, S., and S. Hekman. 2008. "Introduction: Emerging Models of Materiality in Feminist Theory." In *Material Feminisms*, edited by S. Alaimo and S. Hekman, 1–22. Bloomington: Indiana University Press.

Allen, N., and S. T. Benninghoff. 2004. "TPC Program Snapshots: Developing Curricula and Addressing Challenges." *Technical Communication Quarterly* 13: 157–85. DOI: 10.1207/s15427625tcq1302_3.

Armstrong, J., M. Toscano, N. Kotchko, S. Friedman, M. D. Schwartz, K. S. Virgo, K. Lynch, et al. 2015. "Utilization and Outcomes of *BRCA* Genetic Testing and Counseling in a National Commercially Insured Population: The ABOUT Study." *JAMA Oncology* 1 (9): 1251–60.

Atkinson, S., B. Evans, A. Woods, and R. Kearns. 2015. "'The Medical' and 'Health' in Critical Medical Humanities." *Journal of Medical Humanities* 36:71–81.

Barad, K. 2003. "Posthumanist Performativity: Toward an Understanding of How Matter Comes to Matter." *Signs* 40 (1): 801–31.

———. 2007. *Meeting the Universe Halfway: Quantum Physics and the Entanglement of Matter and Meaning.* Durham, NC: Duke University Press.

Barnett, S., and C. Boyle, eds. 2016. *Rhetoric, through Everyday Things.* Tuscaloosa: University of Alabama Press.

Barthes, R. 1986. *The Rustle of Language.* New York: Hill and Wang.

Barton, E. 2004. "Discourse Methods and Critical Practice in Professional Communication: The Front-Stage and Back-Stage Discourse of Prognosis in Medicine." *Journal of Business and Technical Communication* 18 (1): 67–111.

Barton, E., and R. Marback. 2008. "The Rhetoric of Hope in the Genre of Prognosis." In *Rhetoric of Healthcare: Essays toward a New Disciplinary Inquiry*, edited by B. Heifferon and S. C. Brown, 15–32. Cresskill, NJ: Hampton Press.

Bateson, M. C. 1994. *Peripheral Visions: Learning along the Way.* New York: Harper Collins Publishers.

Beck, Ulrich. 1999. *World Risk Society.* Cambridge: Polity Press.

Belling, C. 2010. "Narrating Oncogenesis: The Problem of Telling When Cancer Begins." *Narrative* 18 (2): 229–47.

Bennett, J. 2010. *Vibrant Matter: A Political Ecology of Things*. Durham, NC: Duke University Press.

Berg, M. 1998. *Differences in Medicine: Unraveling Practices, Techniques, and Bodies*. Durham, N.C.: Duke University Press.

Berlant, L. G. 2011. *Cruel Optimism*. Durham, NC: Duke University Press.

Bernstein, P. L. 2003. "The Failure of Invariance." In *The Handbook of Risk*, edited by B. Warwick, 3–16. Hoboken, NJ: John Wiley and Sons.

Bero, L., and D. Rennie. 1995. "The Cochrane Collaboration: Preparing, Maintaining, and Disseminating Systematic Reviews of the Effects of Health Care." *Journal of the American Medical Association* 274 (24): 1935–38.

Bianconi, E., A. Piovesan, F. Facchin, A. Beraudi, R. Casadei, F. Frabetti, et al. 2013. "An Estimation of the Number of Cells in the Human Body." *Annals of Human Biology* 40 (6): 463–71.

Bland, J. M., and D. G. Altman. 1995. "Multiple Significance Tests: The Bonferroni Method." *BMJ* 310 (6973): 170.

Bogost, I. 2007. *Persuasive Games: The Expressive Power of Videogames*. Cambridge, MA: MIT Press.

Bohm, D. 1981. *Wholeness and the Implicate Order*. London: Routledge and Kegan Paul.

Bowker, G., and S. L. Star. 1999. *Sorting Things Out: Classification and Its Consequences*. Cambridge, MA: MIT Press.

Braidotti, R. 2007. "Feminist Epistemology after Postmodernism: Critiquing Science, Technology and Globalisation." *Interdisciplinary Science Reviews* 32 (1): 65–74.

———. 2013. *The Posthuman*. Malden, MA: Polity Press.

Bram, U. 2014. *Thinking Statistically*. Charleston, NC: Kuri Books.

Brock, K. 2012. "One Hundred Thousand Billion Processes: Oulipian Computation and the Composition of Digital Cybertexts." *Technoculture*, vol. 2. http://tcjournal.org/drupal/vol2/brock.

———. 2014. "Enthymeme as Rhetorical Algorithm." *Present Tense* 4 (1): 1–7.

Brown, J. 2015. "Being Cellular Race, the Inhuman, and the Plasticity of Life." *GLQ: A Journal of Lesbian and Gay Studies* 21 (2–3): 321–41.

Brown, J. J., Jr. 2014. "The Machine That Therefore I Am." *Philosophy and Rhetoric* 47 (4): 494–514.

Brown, W. 2015. *Undoing the Demos: Neoliberalism's Stealth Revolution*. Cambridge, MA: MIT Press.

Buehl, J. 2016. *Assembling Arguments: Multimodal Rhetoric and Scientific Discourse*. Columbia: University of South Carolina Press.

Buguliskis, J. S. 2015. "The Big Data Addiction—NGS Has It Bad." *Genetic Engineering and Biotechnology News*, May 6. http://www.genengnews.com/insight-and-intelligence/the-big-data-addiction-ngs-has-it-bad/77900442/.

Burnyeat, M. F. 1996. "Enthymeme: Aristotle on the Rationality of Rhetoric." In *Essays on Aristotle's Rhetoric*, edited by A. O. Rorty, 88–115. Berkeley: University of California Press.

Busch, L. 2011. *Standards: Recipes for Reality.* Cambridge, MA: MIT Press.

Butler, J. 1994. "Contingent Foundations: Feminism and the Question of 'Postmodernism.'" In *The Postmodern Turn: New Perspectives on Social Theory,* edited by S. Seidman, 153–70. New York: Cambridge University Press.

———. 2006. *Precarious Life: The Powers of Mourning and Violence.* Brooklyn, NY: Verso.

Callon, M., P. Lascoumes, and Y. Barthe. 2009. *Acting in an Uncertain World: An Essay on Technical Democracy.* Translated by G. Burchell. Cambridge, MA: MIT Press.

Cappelleri, J. C., K. H. Zou, A. G. Bushmakin, J. M. J. Alvir, D. Alemayehu, and T. Symonds. 2013. *Patient-Reported Outcomes: Measurement, Implementation and Interpretation.* Boca Raton, FL: CRC Press.

Cartright, L. 1995. *Screening the Body: Tracing Medicine's Visual Culture.* Minneapolis: University of Minnesota Press.

Ceccarelli, L. 2001. *Shaping Science with Rhetoric: The Cases of Dobzhansky, Schrodinger, and Wilson.* Chicago: University of Chicago Press.

Center for Disease Control and Prevention. 2015. "Genomic Testing." Last updated November 18, 2015. http://www.cdc.gov/genomics/gtesting/index.htm.

Chalmers, I., K. Dickersin, P. Glasziou, M. Gray, G. Guyatt, B. Haynes, D. Rennie, D. L. Sackett, and R. Smith. 2014. *Evidence-Based Medicine: An Oral History Video.* Chicago: American Medical Association. http://ebm.jamanetwork.com/.

Charles, C., A. Gafni, and T. Whelan. 1997. "Shared Decision-Making in the Medical Encounter: What Does It Mean? (Or, It Takes at Least Two to Tango)." *Social Science and Medicine* 44 (5): 681–92.

———. 1999. "Decision-Making in the Physician-Patient Encounter: Revisiting the Shared Treatment Decision-Making Model." *Social Science and Medicine* 49 (5): 651–61.

Charon, R., and P. Wyer. 2008. "Narrative Evidence Based Medicine." *Lancet* 371 (9609): 296–97.

Chen, Caroline. 2015. "Color Genomics Sells $249 Breast Cancer Gene Test to Masses." *Bloomberg Business.* April 20. http://www.bloomberg.com/news/articles/2015-04-21/color-genomics-brings-245-breast-cancer-risk-test-kit-to-masses.

Clarke, A. 2005. *Situational Analysis: Grounded Theory after the Postmodern Turn.* Thousand Oaks, CA: Sage.

Clarke, A. E., J. K. Shim, L. Mamo, J. R. Fosket, and J. R. Fishman. 2010. *Biomedicalization: Technoscience, Health, and Illness in the US.* Durham, NC: Duke University Press.

Cochrane, A. L. 1972. *Effectiveness and Efficiency: Random Reflections on Health Services.* London: Nuffield Provincial Hospitals Trust.

Cochrane Community. 2013. "Chronology of Significant Events and Milestones in Cochrane's History." Archive of the Old Cochrane Community Site. Updated December 12, 2013. http://community-archive.cochrane.org/about-us/history.

Cohen, J. 1964. *Behaviour in Uncertainty and Its Social Implications*. Oxford: Basic Books.

Cohen, J., and A. Meskin. 2004. "On the Epistemic Value of Photographs." *Journal of Aesthetics and Art Criticism* 62:197–210.

Cohen, P. R., D. Day, J. De Lisio, M. Greenberg, R. Kjeldsen, D. Suthers, and P. Berman. 1987. "Management of Uncertainty in Medicine." *International Journal of Approximate Reasoning* 1 (1): 103–16.

Collins, H., and T. Pinch. 2008. *Dr. Golem: How to Think about Medicine*. Chicago: University of Chicago Press.

Color Genomics. 2016. "Hereditary Cancer Genetic Test." White Paper. April 28. https://s3.amazonaws.com/color-static-prod/pdfs/validationWhitePaper.pdf.

Condit, C. M. 1996. "How Bad Science Stays That Way: Brain Sex, Demarcation, and the Status of Truth in the Rhetoric of Science." *Rhetoric Society Quarterly* 26 (4): 83–109.

———. 1999. *The Meanings of the Gene: Public Debates about Human Heredity*. Madison: University of Wisconsin Press.

———. 2013. "'Mind the Gaps': Hidden Purposes and Missing Internationalism in Scholarship on the Rhetoric of Science and Technology in Public Discourse." *Poroi* 9 (1): 3.

Connolly, W. E. 2013. *The Fragility of Things*. Durham, NC: Duke University Press.

D'Agostino, R. B., Sr. 2011. "Changing Endpoints in Breast-Cancer Drug Approval — the Avastin Story." *New England Journal of Medicine* 365 (2): e2.

Dahl, M. 2016. "The Psychology of 'Unnecessary' Mastectomies." *Science of Us* (blog). *New York*. March 15. http://nymag.com/scienceofus/2016/03/the-psychology-of-unnecessary-mastectomies.html.

Danius, S. 2002. *The Senses of Modernism: Technology, Perception, and Aesthetics*. Ithaca, NY: Cornell University Press.

Daston, L. 2000. *Biographies of Scientific Objects*. Chicago: University of Chicago Press.

Davies, H. T., and I. K. Crombie. 2009. *What Are Confidence Intervals and p-Values?* London: Hayward Medical Communications.

Davis, D. 2005. "Addressing Alterity: Rhetoric, Hermeneutics, and the Nonappropriative Relation." *Philosophy and Rhetoric* 38 (3): 191–212.

Dawson, M. J. 2013. *Paul Lauterbur and the Invention of MRI*. Cambridge, MA: MIT Press.

Day, R. E. 2014. *Indexing It All: The [Subject] in the Age of Documentation, Information, and Data*. Cambridge, MA: MIT Press.

Deleuze, G., and F. Guattari. 1987. *A Thousand Plateaus*. Translated by B. Massumi. Minneapolis: University of Minnesota Press.

Denny, K. 1999. "Evidence-Based Medicine and Medical Authority." *Journal of Medical Humanities* 20 (4): 247–63.

Derkatch, C. 2008. "Method as Argument: Boundary Work in Evidence-Based Medicine." *Social Epistemology* 22 (4): 371–88.

*References*

———. 2016. *Bounding Biomedicine: Evidence and Rhetoric in the New Science of Alternative Medicine.* Chicago: University of Chicago Press.

Dixon-Woods, M., S. Bonas, A. Booth, D. R. Jones, T. Miller, A. J. Sutton, et al. 2006. "How Can Systematic Reviews Incorporate Qualitative Research? A Critical Perspective." *Qualitative Research* 6 (1): 27–44.

Dolmage, J. 2009. "Metis, Mêtis, Mestiza, Medusa: Rhetorical Bodies across Rhetorical Traditions." *Rhetoric Review* 28 (1): 1–28.

Dourish, P. 2004. *Where the Action Is: The Foundations of Embodied Interaction.* Cambridge, MA: MIT Press.

Dourish, P., and G. Bell. 2011. *Divining a Digital Future: Mess and Mythology in Ubiquitous Computing.* Cambridge, MA: MIT Press.

Druss, B. G., and S. C. Marcus. 2005. "Growth and Decentralization of the Medical Literature: Implications for Evidence-Based Medicine." *Journal of the Medical Library Association* 93 (4): 499.

Dumit, J. 2004. *Picturing Personhood: Brain Scans and Biomedical Identity.* Princeton, NJ: Princeton University Press.

Dunmire, P. L. 2010. "Knowing and Controlling the Future: A Review of Futurology." *Prose Studies* 32 (3): 240–63.

Edbauer, J. 2005. "Unframing Models of Public Distribution: From Rhetorical Situation to Rhetorical Ecologies." *Rhetoric Society Quarterly* 35 (4): 5–24.

Elkins, J. 1996. *The Object Stares Back: On the Nature of Seeing.* San Diego, CA: Simon and Schuster.

Engeström, Y. 1993. "Developmental Studies of Work as a Testbench of Activity Theory: The Case of Primary Care Medical Practice." In *Understanding Practice: Perspectives on Activity and Context,* edited by S. Chaiklin and J. Lave, 64–103. Cambridge: Cambridge University Press.

———. 2001. "Making Expansive Decisions: An Activity-Theoretical Study of Practitioners Building Collaborative Medical Care for Children." In *Decision Making: Social and Creative Dimensions,* edited by C. M. Allwood and M. Selart, 281–301. Berlin: Springer Science and Business Media.

———. 2006. "Development, Movement and Agency: Breaking Away into Mycorrhizae Activities." In *Building Activity Theory in Practice: Toward the Next Generation,* edited by K. Yamazumi, 1:1–46. Osaka: Center for Human Activity Theory, Kansai University.

Eskin, C. R. 2002. "Hippocrates, Kairos, and Writing in the Sciences." In *Rhetoric and Kairos: Essays in History, Theory, and Praxis,* edited by P. Sipiora and J. S. Bamlin, 97–113. Albany: State University of New York Press.

"Fact Sheet: President Obama's Precision Medicine Initiative." 2015. Press release, Office of the Press Secretary, The White House. January 30. https://www.whitehouse.gov/the-press-office/2015/01/30/fact-sheet-president-obama-s-precision-medicine-initiative.

Fahnestock, J. 1986. "Accommodating Science: The Rhetorical Life of Scientific Facts." *Written Communication* 3 (3): 275–96.

Fahnestock, J., and M. Secor. 1988. "The Stases in Scientific and Literary Argument." *Written Communication* 5 (4): 427–43.

Fallowfield, L. J., and A. Fleissig. 2012. "The Value of Progression-Free Survival to Patients with Advanced-Stage Cancer." *Nature Reviews Clinical Oncology* 9 (1): 41–47.

Farkas, K., and C. Haas. 2012. "A Grounded Theory Approach for Studying Writing and Literacy." In *Practicing Research in Writing Studies: Reflexive and Ethically Responsible Research*, edited by K. M. Powell and P. Takayoshi, 81–96. New York: Hampton Press.

Feinstein, A. R. 1973. "An Analysis of Diagnostic Reasoning. I. The Domains and Disorders of Clinical Macrobiology." *Yale Journal of Biology and Medicine* 46 (3): 212.

Ferlay, J., I. Soerjomataram, M. Ervik, R. Dikshit, S. Eser, C. Mathers, M. Rebelo, D. M. Parkin, D. Forman, and F. Bray. "GLOBOCAN 2012 v1.0, Cancer Incidence and Mortality Worldwide: IARC CancerBase No. 11." International Agency for Research on Cancer, Lyon, France. Accessed January 16, 2015. http://globocan .iarc.fr.

Fisher, R. A. 1921. "Studies in Crop Variation. I. An Examination of the Yield of Dressed Grain from Broadbalk." *Journal of Agricultural Science* 11 (2): 107–35.

Fleck, L. 1977. *Genesis and Development of a Scientific Fact*. Chicago: University of Chicago Press.

Fountain, T. K. 2014. *Rhetoric in the Flesh: Trained Vision, Technical Expertise, and the Gross Anatomy Lab*. New York: Routledge.

Frank, P. 2015. "UCLA's Medical School's 'Guest Artist' Is Helping to Teach Doctors about Disease." *Huffington Post*. May 20. http://www.huffingtonpost.com/2015 /05/20/ted-meyer-geffen-medical-school_n_7325072.html.

French, R. 2003. *Medicine before Science: The Rational and Learned Doctor from the Middle Ages to the Enlightenment*. Cambridge: Cambridge University Press.

Frost, S. 2011. "The Implications of the New Materialisms for Feminist Epistemology." In *Feminist Epistemology and Philosophy of Science: Power in Knowledge*, edited by H. E. Grasswick, 69–83. New York: Springer.

Gage, J. T. 1991. "A General Theory of the Enthymeme for Advanced Composition." In *Teaching Advanced Composition: Why and How*, edited by K. H. Adams and J. L. Adams, 161–78. Portsmouth, NH: Boynton/Cook.

Garcia, A. 2010. *The Pastoral Clinic: Addiction and Dispossession along the Rio Grande*. Berkeley: University of California Press.

Garrison, K. 2007. "The Personal Is Rhetorical: War, Protest, and Peace in Breast Cancer Narratives." *Disability Studies Quarterly* 27 (4). http://dsq-sds.org /article/view/52/52.

Gatens, M. 1996. *Imaginary Bodies: Ethics, Power and Corporeality*. New York: Routledge.

GATK. 2012. *The GATK Guide Book*. Version 2.7-4. Cambridge, MA: Broad Institute.

https://www.broadinstitute.org/gatk/guide/pdfdocs/GATK_GuideBook_2.7-4
.pdf.

Gawande, A. 2014. "The Best Possible Day." *New York Times*, October 4. http://www
.nytimes.com/2014/10/05/opinion/sunday/the-best-possible-day.html?_r=0.

Gieryn, T. F. 1999. *Cultural Boundaries of Science: Credibility on the Line.* Chicago:
University of Chicago Press.

Glaser, B. G., and A. L. Strauss. 1965. *Awareness of Dying.* New Brunswick, NJ:
Aldine Transaction.

———. (1967) 2007. *The Discovery of Grounded Theory: Strategies for Qualitative
Research.* New Brunswick, NJ: Aldine Transaction.

Goffman, E. 1959. *The Presentation of Self in Everyday Life.* Garden City, NY:
Anchor.

Gorman, M. E. 2002. "Levels of Expertise and Trading Zones: A Framework for
Multidisciplinary Collaboration." *Social Studies of Science* 32 (5–6): 933–38.

Gøtzsche, P. C., O. J. Hartling, M. Nielsen, and J. Brodersen. 2009. "Screening for
Breast Cancer with Mammography." Nordic Cochrane Centre. http://nordic
.cochrane.org/sites/nordic.cochrane.org/files/uploads/images/mammography
/mammography-leaflet.pdf.

Gøtzsche, P. C., and K. J. Jørgensen. 2013. "Screening for Breast Cancer with
Mammography: A Review." Cochrane Library. June 4. http://www.cochrane.org
/CD001877/BREASTCA_screening-for-breast-cancer-with-mammography.

Graham, S. S. 2011. "Dis-ease or Disease? Ontological Rarefaction in the Medical-
Industrial Complex." *Journal of Medical Humanities* 32 (3): 167–86.

Graham, S. S., and C. Herndl. 2013. "Multiple Ontologies in Pain Management:
Toward a Postplural Rhetoric of Science." *Technical Communication Quarterly*
22 (2): 103–25.

Greenhalgh, T. 2012. "Why Do We Always End Up Here? Evidence-Based Medicine's
Conceptual Cul-de-Sacs and Some Off-Road Alternative Routes." *Journal of
Primary Healthcare* 4 (2): 92–97.

Greenhalgh, T., J. Howick, and N. Maskrey. 2014. "Evidence-Based Medicine: A
Movement in Crisis?" *The BMJ.* June 13. DOI: http://dx.doi.org/10.1136/bmj
.g3725.

Greenhalgh, T., and J. Russell. 2006. "Reframing Evidence Synthesis as Rhetorical
Action in the Policy Making Drama." *Healthcare Policy* 1 (2): 34.

Gries, L. 2015. *Still Life with Rhetoric: A New Materialist Approach for Visual
Rhetorics.* Boulder: University Press of Colorado.

Grossman, J., and J. Leach. 2008. "The Rhetoric of Research Methodology." *Social
Epistemology* 22 (4): 325–31.

Grosz, E. 1994. *Volatile Bodies: Toward a Corporeal Feminism.* Bloomington: Indiana
University Press.

———. 2004. *The Nick of Time: Politics, Evolution, and the Untimely.* Durham, NC:
Duke University Press.

Grusin, R. 2015. *The Nonhuman Turn*. Minneapolis: University of Minnesota Press.

Guattari, F. 1995. *Chaosmosis: An Ethico-Aesthetic Paradigm*. Bloomington: Indiana University Press.

Guyatt, G., A. D. Oxman, E. A. Akl, R. Kunz, G. Vist, J. Brozek, S. Norris et al. 2011. "GRADE Guidelines: 1. Introduction—GRADE Evidence Profiles and Summary of Findings Tables." *Journal of Clinical Epidemiology* 64 (4): 383–94.

Guyatt, G. H., A. D. Oxman, G. E. Vist, R. Kunz, Y. Falck-Ytter, P. Alonso-Coello, and H. J. Schünemann. 2008. "GRADE: An Emerging Consensus on Rating Quality of Evidence and Strength of Recommendations." *BMJ* 336 (7650): 924–26.

Haas, C., and S. P. Witte. 2001. "Writing as an Embodied Practice: The Case of Engineering Standards." *Journal of Business and Technical Communication* 15 (4): 413–57.

Hacking, I. 1975. *The Emergence of Probability: A Philosophical Study of Early Ideas about Probability, Induction and Statistical Inference*. New York: Cambridge University Press.

Haghighian, N. S. 2006. "Natascha Sadr Haghighian's Proposal for *Signing Microscope, 2005*." In *Sensorium: Embodied Experience, Technology, and Contemporary Art*, edited by C. A. Jones, 67. Cambridge, MA: MIT Press.

Hairston, M. C. 1986. "Bringing Aristotle's Enthymeme into the Composition Classroom." In *Rhetoric and Praxis: The Contribution of Classical Rhetoric to Practical Reasoning*, edited by J. D. Moss, 59–77. Washington, DC: Catholic University of America Press.

Happe, K. E. 2013. *The Material Gene: Gender, Race, and Heredity after the Human Genome Project*. New York: New York University Press.

Haraway, D. J. 1988. "Situated Knowledges: The Science Question in Feminism and the Privilege of Partial Perspective." *Feminist Studies* 14 (3): 575–99.

———. 1991. *Simians, Cyborgs, and Women: The Reinvention of Women*. New York: Routledge.

———. 1997. *Modest_Witness@Second_Millennium. FemaleMan_Meets_Onco Mouse: Feminism and Technoscience*. New York: Routledge.

———. 2008. *When Species Meet*. Minneapolis: University of Minnesota Press.

Harding, S. 2006. *Science and Social Inequality: Feminist and Postcolonial Issues*. Urbana-Champaign: University of Illinois Press.

Harris, O. J., and J. Robb. 2012. "Multiple Ontologies and the Problem of the Body in History." *American Anthropologist* 114 (4): 668–79.

Hawhee, D. 2002. "Kairotic Encounters." *Tennessee Studies in Literature* 39:16–35.

Haynes, P. 2014. "Review: Tracey Sarsfield's Reflected Exhibition 'Elegant and Eloquent' Study of Relationships." *Canberra Times*. August 12. http://www .canberratimes.com.au/national/review-tracey-sarsfields-reflected-exhibition -elegant-and-eloquent-study-of-relationships-20140811-102rae.html.

Heard, M. M. 2013. "Tonality and *Ethos*." *Philosophy and Rhetoric* 46 (1): 44–64.

Heeßel, N. P. 2004. "Diagnosis, Divination and Disease: Towards an Understanding of the Rationale behind the Babylonian Diagnostic Handbook." In *Magic and*

*Rationality in Ancient Near Eastern and Graeco-Roman Medicine*, edited by H. F. J. Horfstmanshoff and M. Stol, 97–116. Boston: Brill.

Heidegger, M. 1971. *Poetry, Language, Thought.* Translated by A. Hofstadter. New York: Harper and Row.

———. 1977. *The Question Concerning Technology and Other Essays.* Translated by William Lovitt. New York: Harper Torchbooks.

Hekman, S. 2008. "Constructing the Ballast: An Ontology for Feminism." In *Material Feminisms*, edited by S. Alaimo and S. Hekman, 85–119. Bloomington: Indiana University Press.

Higgins, J. P. T., and S. Green, eds. 2005. *Cochrane Handbook for Systematic Reviews of Interventions.* Version 4.2.5. Chichester: John Wiley & Sons.

———. 2008. *Cochrane Handbook for Systematic Reviews of Interventions.* Version 5.0.0. Chichester: Wiley-Blackwell.

———. 2011. *Cochrane Handbook for Systematic Reviews of Interventions.* Version 5.1.0. Hoboken, NJ: Wiley. www.cochrane-handbook.org.

Higgins, J. P., S. G. Thompson, J. J. Deeks, and D. G. Altman. 2003. "Measuring Inconsistency in Meta-Analyses." *BMJ* 327 (7414): 557–60.

Hikins, J. and R. Cherwitz. 2011. "On the Ontological and Epistemological Dimensions of Expertise: Why 'Reality' and 'Truth' Matter and How We Might Find Them." *Social Epistemology* 25 (3): 291–308.

Hollenberg, N. K., V. J. Dzau, and G. H. Williams. 1980. Reply to H. Sacks, S. Kupfer, and T. C. Chalmers, "Are Uncontrolled Clinical Studies Ever Justified?" *New England Journal of Medicine* 303:1067.

Hughes, E. C. 1971. *The Sociological Eye.* Chicago: Aldine-Atherton.

Hyde, M. J. 2011. "The Expertise of Human Beings and Depression." *Social Epistemology* 25 (3): 263–74.

Ihde, D. 2002. *Bodies in Technology.* Minneapolis: University of Minnesota Press.

Ilic, D., M. M Neuberger, M. Djulbegovic, and P. Dahm. 2013. "Screening for Prostate Cancer." January 31. http://onlinelibrary.wiley.com/doi/10.1002/14651858.CD004720.pub3/full.

Iliopoulos, C. S., D. Kourie, L. Mouchard, T. K. Musombuka, S. P. Pissis, and C. de Ridder. 2012. "An Algorithm for Mapping Short Reads to a Dynamically Changing Genomic Sequence." *Journal of Discrete Algorithms* 10:15–22.

Illich, I. 1981. *Shadow Work.* Boston: Marion Boyars.

Illumina, Inc. 2016. "Next-Generation Sequencing (NGS)." http://www.illumina.com/technology/next-generation-sequencing.html.

Ingold, T. 2000. *The Perception of the Environment: Essays on Livelihood, Dwelling and Skill.* London: Routledge.

Institute of Medicine (US). Committee on Quality of Health Care in America. 2001. *Crossing the Quality Chasm: A New Health System for the 21st Century.* Washington, DC: National Academy Press.

Jain, S. L. 2007. "Living in Prognosis: Toward an Elegiac Politics." *Representations* 98 (1): 77–92.

———. 2013. *Malignant: How Cancer Becomes Us*. Berkeley: University of California Press.

Jasanoff, S. 2003. "Technologies of Humility: Citizen Participation in Governing Science." *Minerva* 41 (3): 223–44.

———. 2004. *States of Knowledge: The Co-Production of Science and the Social Order*. New York: Routledge.

Jemal, A., F. Bray, M. M. Center, J. Ferlay, E. Ward, and D. Forman. 2011. "Global Cancer Statistics." *CA: A Cancer Journal for Clinicians* 61 (2): 69–90.

Jolie, A. 2013. "My Medical Choice." *New York Times*, May 14. http://www.nytimes .com/2013/05/14/opinion/my-medical-choice.html?_r=0.

Jones, N. B., J. Wilson, L. Kotur, J. Stephens, W. B. Farrar, and D. M. Agnese. 2009. "Contralateral Prophylactic Mastectomy for Unilateral Breast Cancer: An Increasing Trend at a Single Institution." *Annals of Surgical Oncology* 16 (10): 2691–96.

Kahneman, D., and A. Tversky. 1984. "Choices, Values, and Frames." *American Psychologist* 39 (4): 341–50.

Keller, E. F. 2009. *Making Sense of Life: Explaining Biological Development with Models, Metaphors, and Machines*. Cambridge, MA: Harvard University Press.

Kennedy, K. 2010. "Textual Machinery: Authorial Agency and Bot-Written Texts in Wikipedia." In *The Responsibilities of Rhetoric*, edited by M. Smith and B. Warnick, 303–9. Long Grove, IL: Waveland.

King, D. 1995. "The State of Eugenics." *New Statesman and Society* 8:25–26.

Klaver, E. 2009. *The Body in Medical Culture*. Albany: State University of New York Press.

Knorr Cetina, K. 2009. *Epistemic Cultures: How the Sciences Make Knowledge*. Cambridge, MA: Harvard University Press.

———. 2013. *The Manufacture of Knowledge: An Essay on the Constructivist and Contextual Nature of Science*. New York: Pergamon Press.

Knox, R. 2011. "Avastin as Breast Cancer Treatment Tests FDA's Ability to Say No." *Shots: Health News from NPR*. NPR, June 29. http://www.npr.org/sections/health -shots/2011/06/29/137493653/avastin-as-breast-cancer-treatment-tests-fdas -ability-to-say-no.

Kramer, A. 2015. "The Genomic Imaginary: Genealogical Heritage and the Shaping of Bioconvergent Identities." *MediaTropes* 5 (1): 80–104.

Kress, G., and T. van Leeuwen. 2006. *Reading Images: The Grammar of Visual Design*. 2nd ed. New York: Routledge.

Kulvicki, J. 2010. "Knowing with Images: Medium and Message." *Philosophy of Science* 77:295–313.

Kurian, A. W., D. Y. Lichtensztajn, T. H. Keegan, D. O. Nelson, C. A. Clarke, and S. L. Gomez. 2014. "Use of and Mortality after Bilateral Mastectomy Compared with Other Surgical Treatments for Breast Cancer in California, 1998–2011." *Journal of the American Medical Association* 312 (9): 902–14.

Kuriyama, S. 1999. *The Expressiveness of the Body and the Divergence of Greek and Chinese Medicine.* New York: Zone Books.

Lambert, H. 2006. "Accounting for EBM: Notions of Evidence in Medicine." *Social Science and Medicine* 62 (11): 2633–45.

Lampland, M., and S. L. Star. 2009. *Standards and Their Stories: How Quantifying, Classifying, and Formalizing Practices Shape Everyday Life.* Ithaca, NY: Cornell University Press.

Landecker, H. 2002. "New Times for Biology: Nerve Cultures and the Advent of Cellular Life In Vitro." *Studies in History and Philosophy of Science Part C: Studies in History and Philosophy of Biological and Biomedical Sciences* 33 (4): 667–94.

———. 2004. "Building 'A New Type of Body in Which to Grow a Cell': Tissue Culture at the Rockefeller Institute, 1910–1914." In *Creating a Tradition of Biomedical Research Contributions to the History of the Rockefeller University,* edited by D. H. Stapleton, 135–50. New York: Rockefeller University Press.

———. 2007. *Culturing Life: How Cells Became Technologies.* Cambridge, MA: Harvard University Press.

Latour, B. 1987. *Science in Action: How to Follow Scientists and Engineers through Society.* Cambridge, MA: Harvard University Press.

———. 1992. "Where Are the Missing Masses? The Sociology of a Few Mundane Artifacts." In *Shaping Technology/Building Society: Studies in Sociotechnical Change,* edited by W. Bijker and J. Law, 225–58. Cambridge, MA: MIT Press.

———. 1993. *The Pasteurization of France.* Cambridge, MA: Harvard University Press.

———. 2005. *Reassembling the Social: An Introduction to Actor-Network-Theory.* Oxford: Oxford University Press.

Latour, B., and S. Woolgar. 1986. *Laboratory Life: The Construction of Scientific Facts.* Princeton, NJ: Princeton University Press.

Leander, N. B. 2008. "To Begin with the Beginning: Birth, Origin, and Narrative Inception." In *Narrative Beginnings: Theories and Practices,* edited by B. Richardson, 15–28. Lincoln: University of Nebraska Press.

Lee, W. D., J. Drazen, P. A. Sharp, and R. S. Langer. 2013. *From X-Rays to DNA: How Engineering Drives Biology.* Cambridge, MA: MIT Press.

Lefebvre, H. 1974. *The Production of Space.* Translated by Donald Nicholson-Smith. Malden, MA: Blackwell Publishing.

Lippman, A. 1991. "Prenatal Genetic Testing and Screening: Constructing Needs and Reinforcing Inequities." *American Journal of Law and Medicine* 17 (1–2): 15–50.

Little, M., C. F. Jordens, K. Paul, K. Montgomery, and B. Philipson. 1998. "Liminality: A Major Category of the Experience of Cancer Illness." *Social Science and Medicine* 47 (10): 1485–94.

Little, M., C. F. Jordens, K. Paul, E. J. Sayers, J. A. Cruickshank, J. Stegeman, and K. Montgomery. 2002. "Discourse in Different Voices: Reconciling $N = 1$ and $N = $ many." *Social Science and Medicine* 55 (7): 1079–87.

Livingston, J. 2012. *Improvising Medicine: An African Oncology Ward in an Emerging Cancer Epidemic*. Durham, NC: Duke University Press.

Lorde, A. 1980. *The Cancer Journals*. San Francisco: Spinsters.

Lucas, P. J., J. Baird, L. Arai, C. Law, and H. M. Roberts. 2007. "Worked Examples of Alternative Methods for the Synthesis of Qualitative and Quantitative Research in Systematic Reviews." *BMC Medical Research Methodology* 7 (4). http://bmcmedresmethodol.biomedcentral.com/articles/10.1186/1471-2288-7-4.

Lynch, M. 2006. "Discipline and the Material Form of Images: An Analysis of Scientific Visibility." In *Visual Cultures of Science: Rethinking Representational Practices in Knowledge Building and Science Communication*, edited by L. Pauwels, 195–221. Lebanon, NH: University Press of New England.

———. 2013. "Postscript Ontography: Investigating the Production of Things, Deflating Ontology." *Social Studies of Science* 43 (3): 444–62.

Macdonald, R. R. 2004. "Statistical Inference and Aristotle's Rhetoric." *British Journal of Mathematical and Statistical Psychology* 57 (2): 193–203.

Majdik, Z. P., and C. A. Platt. 2012. "Selling Certainty: Genetic Complexity and Moral Urgency in Myriad Genetics' BRAC Analysis Campaign." *Rhetoric Society Quarterly* 42 (2): 120–43.

Majdik, Z. P., and W. M. Keith. 2011. "The Problem of Pluralistic Expertise: A Wittgensteinian Approach to the Rhetorical Basis of Expertise." *Social Epistemology* 25 (3): 275–90.

Manser, R., A. Lethaby, L. B. Irving, C. Stone, G. Byrnes, M. J. Abramson, and D. Campbell. 2013. "Screening for Lung Cancer [Review]." Cochrane Library. http://www.cochrane.org/CD001991/LUNGCA_screening-for-lung-cancer.

Marback, R. 2008. "Unclenching the Fist: Embodying Rhetoric and Giving Objects Their Due." *Rhetoric Society Quarterly* 38 (1): 46–65.

Marks, H. M. 2000. *The Progress of Experiment: Science and Therapeutic Reform in the United States, 1900–1990*. New York: Cambridge University Press.

Massachusetts, and J. B. Davis. 1831. *Report of the Select Committee of the House of Representatives on So Much of the Governor's Speech, at the June Session, 1830, as Relates to Legalizing the Study of Anatomy*. Boston: Dutton and Wentworth, printers to the State.

McGovern, L., J. N. Johnson, R. Paulo, A. Hettinger, V. Singhal, C. Kamath, et al. 2008. "Treatment of Pediatric Obesity: A Systematic Review and Meta-Analysis of Randomized Trials." *Journal of Clinical Endocrinology and Metabolism* 93 (12): 4600–4605.

McNely, B., C. Spinuzzi, and C. Teston. 2015. "Contemporary Research Methodologies in Technical Communication." *Technical Communication Quarterly* 24 (1): 1–13.

McWhorter, L. 1999. *Bodies and Pleasures: Foucault and the Politics of Sexual Normalization*. Bloomington: Indiana University Press.

Mebust, M.R., and S. B. Katz. 2008. "Rhetorical Assumptions, Rhetorical Risks: Communication Models in Genetic Counseling." In *Rhetoric of Healthcare: Essays toward a New Disciplinary Inquiry*, edited by B. Heifferon and S. C. Brown, 91–114. Cresskill, NJ: Hampton Press.

Miles, M. B., and A. M. Huberman. 1994. *Qualitative Data Analysis: An Expanded Sourcebook*. Beverly Hills, CA: Sage.

Miller, C. R. 1994. "Opportunity, Opportunism, and Progress: Kairos in the Rhetoric of Technology." *Argumentation* 8 (1): 81–96.

———. 2003. "The Presumptions of Expertise: The Role of Ethos in Risk Analysis." *Configurations* 11 (2): 163–202.

———. 2010. "Should We Name the Tools? Concealing and Revealing the Art of Rhetoric." In *The Public Work of Rhetoric: Citizen-Scholars and Civic Engagement*, edited by D. Coogan and J. Ackerman, 19–38. Columbia: University of South Carolina Press.

Misra, S., A. Agrawal, W. K. Liao, and A. Choudhary. 2011. "Anatomy of a Hash-Based Long Read Sequence Mapping Algorithm for Next Generation DNA Sequencing." *Bioinformatics* 27 (2): 189–95.

Mol, A. 2002. *The Body Multiple: Ontology in Medical Practice*. Durham, NC: Duke University Press.

Mol, A., and J. Mesman. 1996. "Neonatal Food and the Politics of Theory: Some Questions of Method." *Social Studies of Science* 26 (2): 419–44.

Mol, A., I. Moser, and J. Pols. 2010. *Care in Practice: On Tinkering in Clinics, Homes and Farms*. Bielefeld: Transcript Verlag.

Murray, S. J., and D. L. Steinberg. 2015. "Autopoiesis | Ethopoiesis: Bioconvergent Media in the Age of Neoliberal Biopolitics." *Mediatropes* 5 (1): 125–39.

Mykhalovskiy, E., and L. Weir. 2004. "The Problem of Evidence-Based Medicine: Directions for Social Science. *Social Science and Medicine* 59 (5): 1059–69.

Nadeau, R. 1964. "Hermogenes' *On Stases*: A Translation with an Introduction and Notes." *Speech Monographs* 31 (4): 361–424.

National Comprehensive Cancer Network. (n.d.). "Looking Back on Two Decades of Breast Cancer Treatment: Targeted Therapy and Improved Surgical Procedures Are Key Enhancements." http://www.nccn.org/about/news/newsinfo.aspx?NewsID=491.

Nelson, A. 2008. "Bio Science: Genetic Genealogy Testing and the Pursuit of African Ancestry." *Social Studies of Science* 38:759–83.

Nelson, A., and J. H. Robinson. 2014. "The Social Life of DTC Genetics: The Case of 23andMe." In *Routledge Handbook of Science, Technology and Science*, edited by D. K. Kleinman and K. Moore, 108–23. New York: Routledge.

Northcut, K. M. 2007. "Stasis Theory and Paleontology Discourse." *Writing Instructor*, September.

Nowotny, H. 2007. "How Concepts Behave: The Potential of the Life Sciences and Their Impact on Society." Annual Lecture, Centre for Bioscience, Biomedicine, Biotechnology and Society (BIOS), London School of Economics, June 11.

Nussbaum, M. 1989. *The Fragility of Goodness*. Cambridge: Cambridge University Press.

Olson, D. R. 1996. *The World on Paper: The Conceptual and Cognitive Implications of Writing and Reading.* Cambridge: Cambridge University Press.

O'Rourke, D. H. 2003. "Anthropological Genetics in the Genomic Era: A Look Back and Ahead." *American Anthropologist* 105 (1): 101–9.

Oyama, S., P. Taylor, A. Fogel, R. Lickliter, K. Sterelny, K. C. Smith, and C. van der Weele. 2000. *The Ontogeny of Information: Developmental Systems and Evolution.* Durham, NC: Duke University Press.

Parry, B. 2013. "Knowing Mycellf™: Personalized Medicine and the Economization of Prospective Knowledge about Bodily Fate." In *Knowledge and the Economy*, edited by P. Meusburger, J. Glückler, M. el Meskioui, 157–71. Dordrecht: Springer.

Parthasarathy, S. 2012. *Building Genetic Medicine: Breast Cancer, Technology, and the Comparative Politics of Health Care.* Cambridge, MA: MIT Press.

———. 2014. "Producing the Consumer of Genetic Testing: The Double-Edged Sword of Empowerment." In *Routledge Handbook of Science, Technology, and Society*, edited by D. L. Kleinman and K. Moore, 93–107. New York: Routledge.

Pasveer, B. 2006. "Representing or Mediating: A History and Philosophy of X-Ray Images in Medicine." In *Visual Cultures of Science: Rethinking Representational Practices in Knowledge Building and Science Communication*, edited by L. Pauwels, 41–62. Lebanon, NH: University Press of New England.

Pear, R. 2015. "U.S. Introduces New DNA Standard for Ensuring Accuracy of Genetic Tests." *New York Times*, May 14. http://www.nytimes.com/2015/05/15/health/new-way-to-ensure-accuracy-of-dna-tests-us-announces.html.

Peine, A. 2011. "Challenging Incommensurability: What We Can Learn from Ludwik Fleck for the Analysis of Configurational Innovation." *Minerva* 49 (4): 489–508.

Pender, K. 2012. "Genetic Subjectivity In Situ: A Rhetorical Reading of Genetic Determinism and Genetic Opportunity in the Biosocial Community of FORCE." *Rhetoric and Public Affairs* 15 (2): 319–49.

Perelman, C. 1982. *The Realm of Rhetoric.* Notre Dame, IN: University of Notre Dame Press.

Perelman, C., and L. Olbrechts-Tyteca. 1969. *The New Rhetoric.* Notre Dame, IN: University of Notre Dame Press.

Petticrew, M., and M. Egan. 2006. "Relevance, Rigour and Systematic Reviews." In *Moving beyond Effectiveness in Evidence Synthesis: Methodological Issues in the Synthesis of Diverse Sources of Evidence*, edited by J. Popay, 7–8. London: National Institute for Clinical Excellence.

Phelps, L. W. 1991. *Composition as a Human Science: Contributions to the Self-Understanding of a Discipline.* Oxford: Oxford University Press.

Pickering, A. 1995. *The Mangle of Practice: Time, Agency, and Science.* Chicago: University of Chicago.

Pollack, A. 2010. "FDA Rejects Use of Drug in Cases of Breast Cancer." *New York Times*, December 16.

Popay, J. 2006. "Of Hedgehogs and Foxes: Issues in the Review and Utilisation of

Research-Based Evidence." *International Journal of Evidence-Based Healthcare* 4 (2): 75–76.

Popham, S. L., and S. L. Graham. 2008. "A Structural Analysis of Coherence in Electronic Charts in Juvenile Mental Health." *Technical Communication Quarterly* 17 (2): 149–72.

Porter, T. M. 1996. *Trust in Numbers: the Pursuit of Objectivity in Science and Public Life.* Princeton, NJ: Princeton University Press.

Prelli, L. J. 1989. *A Rhetoric of Science: Inventing Scientific Discourse.* Columbia: University of South Carolina Press.

Prentice, R. 2012. *Bodies in Formation: An Ethnography of Anatomy and Surgery Education.* Durham, NC: Duke University Press.

RevMan. 2011. Review Manager (RevMan) [Computer program]. Version 5.1. Copenhagen: Nordic Cochrane Centre, the Cochrane Collaboration.

Rice, Jeff. 2008. "Urban Mappings: A Rhetoric of the Network." *Rhetoric Society Quarterly* 38 (2): 198–218.

Rich, J. T., J. G. Neely, R. C. Paniello, C. C. Voelker, B. Nussenbaum, and E. W. Wang. 2010. "A Practical Guide to Understanding Kaplan-Meier Curves." *Otolaryngology-Head and Neck Surgery* 143 (3): 331–36.

Richards, S., N. Aziz, S. Bale, D. Bick, S. Das, J. Gastier-Foster, W. W. Grody, et al. 2015. "Standards and Guidelines for the Interpretation of Sequence Variants: A Joint Consensus Recommendation of the American College of Medical Genetics and Genomics and the Association for Molecular Pathology." *Genetics in Medicine* 17 (5): 405–23.

Rickert, T. 2013. *Ambient Rhetoric: The Attunements of Rhetorical Being.* Pittsburgh: University of Pittsburgh Press.

Rogers, E. 1962. *Diffusion of Innovations.* New York: Free Press.

Rotman, B. 2000. *Mathematics as Sign: Writing, Imagining, Counting.* Palo Alto, CA: Stanford University Press.

Saccà, L. 2010. "The Uncontrolled Clinical Trial: Scientific, Ethical, and Practical Reasons for Being." *Internal and Emergency Medicine* 5 (3): 201–4.

Sackett, D. L., W. Rosenberg, J. A. Gray, R. B. Haynes, and W. S. Richardson. 1996. "Evidence Based Medicine: What It Is and What It Isn't." *British Medical Journal* 312 (7023): 71–72.

Sacks, H., S. Kupfer, and T. C. Chalmers. 1980. "Are Uncontrolled Clinical Studies Ever Justified?" *New England Journal of Medicine* 303:1067–67.

Salzberg, S. 2014. "PSA Screening Does More Harm Than Good." *Forbes*, May 19. http://www.forbes.com/sites/stevensalzberg/2014/05/19/psa-screening-does -more-harm-than-good/.

Sauer, B. A. 1998. "Embodied Knowledge: The Textual Representation of Embodied Sensory Information in a Dynamic and Uncertain Material Environment." *Written Communication* 15:131–69. DOI: 10.1177/0741088398015002001.

———. 2003. *The Rhetoric of Risk Technical Documentation in Hazardous Environments.* Mahwah, NJ: L. Erlbaum Associates.

Saunders, B. F. 2010. *CT Suite: The Work of Diagnosis in the Age of Noninvasive Cutting*. Durham, NC: Duke University Press.

Schattner, E. 2015. "On Mammography, Evidence, and Why We Need to Improve Breast Cancer Screening." *Forbes*, April 22. http://www.forbes.com/sites/elaine schattner/2015/04/22/on-mammography-evidence-and-why-we-need-to -improve-breast-cancer-screening/.

Schryer, C. F. 1993. "Records as Genre." *Written Communication* 10 (2): 200–234.

Schryer, C. F., E. Afros, M. Mian, M. Spafford, and L. Lingard. 2009. "The Trial of the Expert Witness Negotiating Credibility in Child Abuse Correspondence." *Written Communication* 26 (3): 215–46.

Schryer, C. F., L. Lingard, M. M. Spafford. 2005. "Techne or Artful Science and the Genre of Case Presentations in Healthcare Settings." *Communication Monographs* 72 (2): 234–60.

Scott, J. B. 2002. "The Public Policy Debate over Newborn HIV Testing: A Case Study of the Knowledge Enthymeme." *Rhetoric Society Quarterly* 32 (2): 57–83.

———. 2006. "Kairos as Indeterminate Risk Management: The Pharmaceutical Industry's Response to Bioterrorism." *Quarterly Journal of Speech* 92 (2): 115–43.

Scribner, S. 1997. *Mind and Social Practice: Selected Writings of Sylvia Scribner*. Cambridge: Cambridge University Press.

Segal, J. Z. 2005. *Health and the Rhetoric of Medicine*. Carbondale: Southern Illinois University Press.

Siebers, T. 2008. "Disability Experience on Trial." In *Material Feminisms*, edited by S. Alaimo and S. Hekman, 291–307. Bloomington: Indiana University Press.

Simmons, W. M., and J. Grabill. 2007. "Toward a Civic Rhetoric for Technologically and Scientifically Complex Places: Invention, Performance, and Participation." *College Composition and Communication* 58 (3): 419–48.

Smith, D. L. 2003. "Intensifying *Phronesis*: Heidegger, Aristotle, and Rhetorical Culture." *Philosophy and Rhetoric* 36 (1): 77–102.

Smith, R., and D. Rennie. 2014. "Evidence-Based Medicine—an Oral History." *Journal of the American Medical Association* 311 (4): 365–67.

Spinuzzi, C. 2003. *Tracing Genres through Organizations: A Sociocultural Approach to Information Design*. Cambridge, MA: MIT Press.

———. 2011. "Losing by Expanding Corralling the Runaway Object." *Journal of Business and Technical Communication* 25 (4): 449–86.

Spinuzzi, C., W. Hart-Davidson, and M. Zachry. 2006. "Chains and Ecologies: Methodological Notes toward a Communicative-Mediational Model of Technologically Mediated Writing." In *Proceedings of the 24th Annual ACM International Conference on Design of Communication*, 43–50. New York: ACM.

Spruance, S. L., J. E. Reid, M. Grace, and M. Samore. 2004. "Hazard Ratio in Clinical Trials." *Antimicrobial Agents and Chemotherapy* 48 (8): 2787–92.

Stafford, B. M. 1993. *Body Criticism: Imaging the Unseen in Enlightenment Art and Medicine*. Cambridge, MA: MIT Press.

Star, S. L. 2010. "This Is Not a Boundary Object: Reflections on the Origin of a Concept." *Science, Technology and Human Values* 35 (5): 601–17.

Star, S. L., and J. R. Griesemer. 1989. "Institutional Ecology, Translations and Boundary Objects: Amateurs and Professionals in Berkeley's Museum of Vertebrate Zoology, 1907–39." *Social Studies of Science* 19 (3): 387–420.

Strauss, A. L. 1987. *Qualitative Analysis for Social Scientists*. Cambridge: Cambridge University Press.

Syverson, Margaret A. 1999. *The Wealth of Reality: An Ecology of Composition*. Carbondale: Southern Illinois University Press.

TallBear, K. 2013. *Native American DNA: Tribal Belonging and the False Promise of Genetic Science*. Minneapolis: University of Minnesota Press.

Teston, C. B. 2009. "A Grounded Investigation of Genred Guidelines in Cancer Care Deliberations." *Written Communication* 26:320–40.

———. 2012a. "Considering Confidentiality in Research Design: Developing Heuristics to Chart the Un-chartable." In *Practicing Research in Writing Studies: Reflections on Ethically Responsible Research*, edited by P. Takayoshi and K. Powell, 303–26. Cresskill, NJ: Hampton Press.

———. 2012b. "Moving from Artifact to Action: A Grounded Investigation of Visual Displays of Evidence during Medical Deliberations." *Technical Communication Quarterly* 21 (3): 187–209.

———. 2016. "Rhetoric, Precarity, and mHealth Technologies." *Rhetoric Society Quarterly* 46 (3): 251–68.

Teston, C., and S. S. Graham. 2012. "Stasis Theory and Meaningful Public Participation in Pharmaceutical Policy-Making." *Present Tense: A Journal of Rhetoric and Society* 2 (2): 1–8.

Teston, C. B., S. S. Graham, R. Baldwinson, A. Li, and J. Swift. 2014. "Public Voices in Pharmaceutical Deliberations: Negotiating 'Clinical Benefit' in the FDA's Avastin Hearing." *Journal of Medical Humanities* 35 (2): 149–70.

Toulmin, S. E. 2003. *The Uses of Argument*. Cambridge: Cambridge University Press.

Toulmin, S. E., R. D. Rieke, and A. Janik. 1984. *An Introduction to Reasoning*. New York: Macmillan.

Tufte, E. R. (1997) 2003. *Visual and Statistical Thinking: Displays of Evidence for Making Decisions*. Cheshire, CT: Graphics Press.

Tuttle, T. M., E. B. Habermann, E. H. Grund, T. J. Morris, and B. A. Virnig. 2007. "Increasing Use of Contralateral Prophylactic Mastectomy for Breast Cancer Patients: A Trend toward More Aggressive Surgical Treatment." *Journal of Clinical Oncology* 25 (33): 5203–9.

Twombly, R. 2011. "Avastin's Uncertain Future in Breast Cancer Treatment." *Journal of the National Cancer Institute* 103 (6): 458–60.

U.S. Food and Drug Administration. 2011. "Hearing on Proposal to Withdraw Approval for Breast Cancer Indication for Bevavizumb (Avastin)." June 28 and 29. http://www.fda.gov/NewsEvents/MeetingsConferencesWorkshops/ucm255874.htm.

*References*　　　　　　　　　　　[ 231

———. 2013. "Warning Letter to 23andMe." November 22. Document no. GEN1300666. Last updated March 28, 2014. http://www.fda.gov/ICECI /EnforcementActions/WarningLetters/2013/ucm376296.htm.

———. 2014. "Accelerated approval." Last updated September 15, 2014. http://www .fda.gov/ForPatients/Approvals/Fast/ucm405447.htm.

———. 2015. "FDA Permits Marketing of First Direct-to-Consumer Genetic Carrier Test for Bloom Syndrome." Press release. http://www.fda.gov/newsevents/news room/pressannouncements/ucm435003.htm.

Van Dijck, J. 2005. *The Transparent Body: A Cultural Analysis of Medical Imaging.* Seattle: University of Washington Press.

Vee, A. 2010. "Proceduracy: Computer Code Writing in the Continuum of Literacy." PhD diss. University of Wisconsin–Madison.

Walsh, L. 2013. *Scientists as Prophets: A Rhetorical Genealogy.* New York: Oxford University Press.

Walsh, L., and K. Walker. 2013. "Uncertainty, Spheres of Argument, and the Transgressive Ethos of the Science Adviser." In *Ethical Issues in Science Communication: A Theory-Based Approach: Proceedings of a Symposium at Iowa State University, May 30–June 1, 2013,* edited by J. Goodwin, M. T. Dahlstrom, and S. Priest, 325–35. Ames, IA: Science Communication Project.

Weinberg, R. A. 2013. *One Renegade Cell: How Cancer Begins.* New York: Basic Books.

Weiser, M. 1991. "The Computer for the 21st Century." *Scientific American* 265 (3): 94–104.

Welhausen, C. A., and R. E. Burnett. 2016. "Visualizing Public Health Risks: Graphical Representations of Smallpox in the Seventeenth, Eighteenth, and Nineteenth Centuries." In *Essays on the History of Statistical Graphics,* edited by C. Kostelnick and M. Kimball, 61–80. Surrey: Ashgate Press.

White, A., and E. Ernst. 2001. "The Case for Uncontrolled Clinical Trials: A Starting Point for the Evidence Base for CAM." *Complementary Therapies in Medicine* 9 (2): 111–16.

Wickman, C. 2012. "Rhetoric, Techné, and the Art of Scientific Inquiry." *Rhetoric Review* 31 (1): 21–40.

Winance, M. 2010. "Care and Disability. Practices of Experimenting, Tinkering with, and Arranging People and Technical Aids." In *Care in Practice: On Tinkering in Clinics, Homes and Farms,* edited by A. Mol, I. Moser, and J. Pols, 93–117. Bielefeld: Transcript Verlag.

Wynn, J. 2009. "Arithmetic of the Species: Darwin and the Role of Mathematics in His Argumentation." *Rhetorica* 27 (1): 76–97.

Ziliak, S. T., and D. N. McCloskey. 2008. "Science Is Judgment, Not Only Calculation: A Reply to Aris Spanos's Review of *The Cult of Statistical Significance.*" *Erasmus Journal for Philosophy and Economics* 1:165–70.

# INDEX

Page numbers followed by *t* indicate a table; those followed by *f* indicate a figure.

bilateral risk-reducing mastectomy, 3–4
biopower, 165–66, 173–75
black box, the, 4, 22
Bland, J. M., 114
Bloom syndrome, 141
body data, 7–8, 33–41; pathology displays of, 8, 33, 36–41; radiology displays of, 8, 34–36; tumor board consideration of, 7–8, 49–52
Bogost, Ian, 139
Bohm, David, 2
Bohr, Niels, 53, 210n3
boundary work, 25, 173–75; boundary infrastructure in, 162–63; boundary objects in, 161–62, 213n17; in genetic testing, 163–68
*Bounding Biomedicine* (Derkatch), 12
Boyle, C., 17–18
BRACAnalysis, 136–37
Braidotti, Rosi, 19, 158
Bram, U., 209n16
BRCA mutations, 3, 134; cancer risk and, 211n1; genetic testing for, 134–37, 141–43, 211n7. *See also* genetic testing
breast cancer, 104t; Angelina Jolie effect and, 3–4, 134, 142, 211n7; bilateral mastectomy for, 3–4, 95; BRCA mutations in, 3, 134, 211n7; CSR on screenings for, 105, 108–12t, 113, 122–26; FDA hearings on Avastin and, 62–68, 88, 91, 122, 208n3, 209n16; genetic testing for, 134–37, 141–43, 211n7; immunotherapies for, 181; potential genetic mutations in, 155; preventive surgeries for, 3–4, 142–43; screening controversies in, 125–26. *See also* Avastin
Brock, K., 139–40
Brown, James J., Jr., 139–40
Brown, Jayna, 56
Brown, Wendy, 160, 213n16

*Building Genetic Medicine* (Parthasarathy), 136
Burnett, R. E., 208n8
Burnyeat, M. F., 78
Busch, L., 130
Butler, Judith, 132

Callon, M., 18, 209n15
cancer: agency of cells of, 55–57, 206n9, 207nn11–12; biopsy of, 34; cellular flux in, 26–27, 205n1; changing standards for treatment of, 95–96; dwelling with disease and, 175–85; hazard rates in, 80, 81, 83–84; in "HeLa" cells, 56; militaristic narratives of, 55, 206n9; overall and progression-free survival rates in, 62, 72, 79f, 80–83; practicing *phronesis* in, 181–82; Precision Medicine Initiative and, 134–35, 149; screening protocols for, 130; staging of, 37, 46, 206n5; standards of care in, 8, 45–46, 130–33; Toulminian analyses of CSRs on, 105, 108–12t, 113, 116–27, 170; tumor board conferences for, 7–8, 27–29, 205nn2–3; uncontrolled trials for, 118–19; visual evidence of, 26–59; worldwide rates of, 104. *See also* randomized, controlled clinical trials (RCTs)
Ceccarelli, L., 213n17
Center for Disease Control and Prevention (CDC), 137
Chalmers, Ian, 99
Chinese medicine, 10–11; twelve pulses of, 16; visual knowledge in, 27
Cicero, 9, 128
Clarke, A.: on actors and actants, 157; on boundary objects, 161; conceptual toolbox of, 146f, 147, 148f; on discourses, 153; situational mapping method of, 25, 144–49, 212n10; on universes of discourses, 158

*Index*

clear margins, 40

cleromancy, 9

clinical trials. *See* randomized, controlled clinical trials (RCTs)

Cochrane, Archie, 97

Cochrane Centre, 97; Archie document repository of, 101; funding of, 99; library of reviews of, 98; RevMan software of, 97, 101, 106

Cochrane Collaboration, 96–99

Cochrane Systematic Review (CSR), 24, 94–103; *Cochrane Handbook* of, 99, 105, 114, 128, 130–31; consensus process in, 101; critiques of, 125–26, 130–33; definition of, 94; dissemination of findings of, 103; flow diagram of, 102*f*; GRADE criteria for, 103*f*, 130; labor of making evidential cuts in, 95–96, 105–6, 113–15, 118–30, 197–203; limitations of, 98–99; origins of, 97–98; planning phase of, 99; PRISMA checklist of, 99, 100*f*, 101–3, 130; publication process of, 103; rhetorical analyses of, 106–15; searching process of, 99, 106; textual features of, 105–6, 107*f*; Toulminian analysis of extratextual features of, 115–30, 170; writing reviews in, 101–3

cohort studies, 121

Collins, H., 172

Color Genomics, 140, 142–43, 149, 211n7; exome sequencing method of, 153–56, 212n14; financial backers of, 158–59; reference materials of, 152; scientific team of, 159

common warrants, 91–92

complex (as term), 205n2

computing evidence, 2, 4, 21–25, 134–68; algorithmic and technical labor of, 138–40, 143, 164–67, 211n3; biopower effects of, 165–66; boundary work in, 162–68; commodification of human

DNA and, 24–25, 135–39, 159; narratives of individual empowerment in, 136, 140–42, 147, 159–60, 163–64, 174–75, 213n16; proprietary techniques in, 139; rhetorical approaches to, 170; rhetorical work of, 139–40, 161–68, 213nn17–20; search and alignment stages of, 153–54; situational mapping of, 25, 144–61, 212n10. *See also* genetic testing; situational mapping of genetic testing

conceptual cul-de-sac, 131–33

confidence intervals, 81, 84–85

Connolly, W., 144

contemporary medical evidence, 11–14

*copia*, 139

coproduction, 11–12, 139, 144, 162

cost-benefit analyses, 208n10

*Cruel Optimism* (Berlant), 181

CSR. *See* Cochrane Systematic Review (CSR)

CT scans, 34, 35

*CT Suite* (Saunders), 52

Dahl, M., 142–43

Darwin, Charles, 91

Davis, D., 176

Day, R. E., 212n13

*De Inventione* (Cicero), 126

Deleuze, Gilles, 18, 175

demographics, 129, 157

Derkatch, C., 12, 131, 161

descriptive studies, 121

diffusion of innovations theory, 210n1

Dixon-Woods, M., et al., 132

DNA profiling, 151–53, 156, 212n11. *See also* genetic testing

Dolmage, J., 177–78

Dourish, P., 92

dwelling, 54–59, 207n10; descriptions of, 176; with disease, 175–85; kairotic attunement in, 58–59, 169

ecological model of rhetoric, 2
Edbauer, Jenny, 2, 15, 20
Edman degradation, 204
*Effectiveness and Efficiency* (Cochrane), 97
effect size, 70*t*, 71, 81, 85–86
Egan, M., 132
Elkins, J., 53
embodied knowledge, 46
Engeström, Y., 72, 143–44
enthymematic reasoning, 77–89, 167, 169–72; definition of, 78; inferential statistics as, 77–89, 93; vs. population-based premises, 172; standard of care documents as, 13–14
environmental pollution, 56, 206n8
eosin Y, 39
episteme, 177
epistemic communities, 91–92
Erasmus, 139
Eskin, C. R., 56
ethic of care, 167–68, 173–75; dwelling with disease in, 175–85; relational well-being in, 174–75
eugenics movement, 137, 212n9
evidence, 1–2, 205n11; algorithmic protocols as, 12–14; black boxes for, 4; in cancer care, 4; clinical trials as, 12, 60–63; in contemporary medicine, 11–14; four kinds of, 2; investigative sites of, 21–23; methods and attunement in, 14–19; navigation of uncertainty in, 1–2; in premodern medicine, 9–11, 205n7; suasive potential of, 16–17, 172. *See also* assessing evidence; computing evidence; synthesizing evidence; visualizing evidence
evidence-based medicine, 5–7, 27, 205n1; Cochrane Systematic Reviews of, 98; on genetic testing, 134–35; methodological rigor of, 5; randomized, controlled clinical trials in, 12,

60–63; rhetorical design of, 5–7; uncontrolled trials and, 118–19
evidencing (as practice), 54
evidential attunement, 14–21, 169–85; ambient attunement in, 17, 138–39; in assessing evidence, 65–67, 88–93, 169–70, 209n16; computational boundary work in, 162–68, 170; in dwelling with disease, 175–85; ethic of care in, 167–68, 173–75; intra-actions in, 19–20; labor of rhetoric in, 20–23, 171–85, 208n7; practicing *phronesis* in, 177–82; role of nonhuman agents in, 17–19; shadow work in, 17–20, 164–66; suasive potential of, 20; in synthesizing evidence, 131–33, 170; with visual evidence, 49–52, 169
exome sequencing, 153–56, 212n14
exons, 154–55

Fahnestock, J., 128, 133, 170
Fallowfield, L. J., 91
Farkas, K., 113
Feinstein, A. R., 14
Ferrier, David, 162
Ferriprox, 68
FISH (fluorescent in situ hybridization) studies, 38–39
Fisher, R. A., 209n16
Fleck, L., 170
Fleckian thought collectives, 132–33
Fleissig, A., 91
Flint (Michigan) water crisis, 174
flux (as concept), 2
Food and Drug Administration (FDA), 23, 208n10; accelerated approval of Avastin by, 60–61, 207n1; Avastin hearing and decision of, 62–68, 88, 91, 208n3, 209n16; definition of "clinical benefit" of, 60; on genetic testing, 137–38, 140–41, 211n4; post-Avastin hearings of, 68–73, 187–96, 208n6,

209n12; probabilistic reasoning of, 73–76; ruling on 23andMe by, 140–41

*Forbes Magazine*, 119

fragility, 182, 213n2

frequentist statistics, 209n13. *See also* inferential statistics

Gage, John, 78

Garrison, K., 55

Gawande, Atul, 63, 92–93

genealogical research, 136, 149

Genentech: Avastin E2100 clinical trial of, 79*f*, 80–88; Avastin hearing of, 60–68, 207n1, 208n3, 209n16; Perjeta hearing of, 72. *See also* Avastin

genetic mutation. *See* mutation

genetic testing, 24–25, 134–68; affordability of, 134–35, 142; algorithmic and technical labor in, 138–40, 143, 164–67, 211n3; Angelina Jolie effect in, 3–4, 134, 142, 211n7; backstage boundary work in, 163–68; biopower effects in, 165–66; for breast cancer, 134–37; consumer risks and, 137–38, 211n2; differing methodologies of, 140, 150–56, 164, 204, 212nn11–14; direct-to-consumer products for, 135–38, 140–43; disclaimer for, 141, 163, 211n5; DNA profiling in, 151–53, 156, 212n11; ethical-ideological consequences of, 136–39, 166–68, 211n2; exome sequencing method of, 153–56, 212n14; for genealogical research, 136, 149; government regulation of, 139, 141, 147, 211nn4–5; marketing of, 136–37, 140–42, 149, 159–60; meaningfulness of, 135; narratives of individual empowerment in, 136, 140–42, 147, 159–60, 163–64, 174–75, 213n16; next-generation genetic sequencing in, 144, 149, 167; patented gene sequences in, 211n7; in precision medicine, 134–

35, 149; profits earned from, 149; reference materials databases in, 151–52, 157–63, 167–68, 213n15; rhetorical work of, 161–68, 170, 213nn17–20; situational analysis of, 144–61, 212n10. *See also* computing evidence; situational mapping of genetic testing

genome, 212n12

genre, 94

Gieryn, T., 8

Glaser, B. G., 29–30, 69

Goody, Jack, 10

Gorman, Michael, 131

Gøtzsche, P. C., 105, 108–12*t*, 122–26

Grabill, J., 90

Graham, S. S., 72–73

Greek premodern medicine, 9–11, 16

Greenhalgh, T., 131–32

Gries, Laurie, 2

Griesemer, J. R., 161

grounded theory method, 29–30, 69, 113, 144

Guattari, Félix, 18–19, 175

Guyatt, Gordon, 5, 97–98, 205n1

Haas, Christina, 7, 46, 113

Hacking, I., 75

Haghighian, N. S., 206n3

Hamburg, Margaret, 62, 208n3

Hanna, Crystal, 60–61, 63, 66, 92

Happe, K. E., 128, 137–38, 143, 206n7

Haraway, Donna: on coproduction and subject-object relationships, 11, 53; on genes, 143, 163; on genetic evidence, 144; on idealized objectivity, 116

Harris, O. J., 17

Hawhee, D., 56

Haynes, Brian, 98

hazard rates, 80, 81, 83–84

Heard, M. M., 176, 178, 181

Heeßel, N. P., 10

Heidegger, Martin, 15, 18, 73, 76, 175–76

Hekman, S., 17, 18, 19–20
hematoxylin, 39
hepatoscopy, 9
HER-2/neu protein, 49
Heraclitus, 2
Hermagoras, 126–28
Hermogenes, 126
Herndl, C., 72–73
high-powered microscopes, 36–37
Hippocrates, 56
Hollenberg, N. K., et al., 119
Homer, 56–57
*homo economicus*, 165
Hood and Hunkapiller method, 204
Howard, Priscilla, 61–63, 66, 92
Howick, J., 132
Huberman, A. M., 69
Human Genome Project (HGP), 137
Huxley, Aldous, 173

*If Body* (Lehrer), 181
Ihde, D., 53
Ilic, D., et al., 105, 108–12*t*, 119–22
Iliopoulos, C. S., et al., 154
Illich, I., 17, 19, 25, 164–66
Illumina, Inc., 149, 160
images. *See* visualizing evidence
immunotherapy, 181
improvisation, 54, 178–79
incommensurability, 72, 89
indeterminacy, 8, 89–90, 210n3
inferential statistics, 65–67, 77–90;
    confidence intervals in, 81, 84–85;
    effect size in, 81, 85–86; enthyme-
    matic premises of, 77–89, 92–93, 167,
    169–70; group means and medians in,
    83–84; hazard rates in, 80, 81, 83–84;
    Kaplan-Meier analysis in, 23, 77–83,
    88; the null hypothesis in, 81–82; ori-
    gins of, 209n16; probabilistic methods
    of, 73–76, 172–73, 209n15; *p* values
    and statistical significance in, 81,
    86–89; statistical power in, 85; sua-

sive qualities of, 74–75, 77; super-
responders and, 66–67, 83–84; time-
based measures in, 83–84; type I
and II errors in, 82–83
Ingold, T., 175–85
*Institutio Oratoria* (Quintilian), 126
interconnectedness, 175
International HapMap Project, 153–54
intra-action, 15, 17, 38–39, 173; agential
    forms of, 19; corporeal-environmental
    forms of, 55; ontological forms of, 161
investigative sites, 21–23

Jain, S. L., 176
Janik, A., 126–27
Jasanoff, Sheila, 11, 144, 163
Jolie, Angelina, 3–4, 134, 142, 211n7
Jørgensen, K. J., 105, 108–12*t*, 122–26

Kahneman, D., 74–75, 76
*kairos*, 23, 28, 52–59, 169
Kaplan, Edward, 79
Kaplan-Meier analysis, 23, 77–83, 88
Keller, Evelyn Fox, 53
Kennedy, K., 139
Knorr Cetina, K., 91, 206n8
Kramer, A., 136, 149, 163
Kuhn, Thomas, 132
Kurian, A. W., et al., 95
Kuriyama, S., 10–11, 16

Lacks, Henrietta, 56
Lampland, M., 17
Landecker, H., 207n12
Lander's technique, 204
Laraki, Othman, 142
Lascoumes, P., 18, 209n15
Latour, B.: on actants and network
    effects, 18, 175, 205n11; on action,
    183; black box construct of, 4; on con-
    structing scientific facts, 17, 134; on
    contexts of discovery, 6; on upstream
    evidential processes, 8

*Index*

pathology imaging (*continued*) frozen sections in, 41–42; high-powered microscopes in, 36–37; material intra-actions in, 37–38; staining in, 39

patient-centered care, 22

patient-reported outcomes (PROs), 90–92

Peckham, Michael, 97

Peginesatide, 69

Pender, K., 159, 166

Perelman, C., 55

Perjeta, 72

PET scans, 35

Petticrew, M., 132

Phelps, L. W., 2, 15

*phronesis*, 21, 23, 25, 167, 177–82; description of, 177–78; in practice, 178–82. *See also* ethic of care

Pickering, A., 18, 175

Pinch, T., 172

Plato, 9

Platt, C. A., 136–37

plus and minus (Sanger) method, 204

*poesis*, 24, 73–76, 90–93, 167, 173, 209n15

pollution, 55, 206n8

Pols, J., 7, 25, 175, 181–82

polymorphisms, 151, 156–58

Porter, T. M., 12, 74

post-Avastin hearings, 68–73, 187–96, 208n6, 209n12

precarity, 24, 179

precision medicine, 24, 167

Precision Medicine Initiative, 134–35, 149, 151*t*, 160

Prelli, L. J., 128

premodern medicine, 2, 9–11, 27, 136, 205n7

probabilistic reasoning, 73–76; material making-power of, 75–76, 172–73; *poesis* of, 24, 73–76, 90–93, 167, 173, 209n15; premodern practices of, 75–

76; suasive qualities of, 74–75, 209n15. *See also* inferential statistics

progression-free survival rates, 62, 72, 79*f*, 80–83

prostate cancer, 104*t*, 105, 108–12*t*, 119–22

"PSA Testing Does More Harm Than Good" (Salzberg), 119

pulse, 10–11, 16

*p* values, 81, 86–89

qualitative evidence, 24, 98, 132–33

quality-of-life (QoL) variables, 90–92, 208n10

Quintilian, 126

radiology images, 34–36; CT scans in, 35; MRIs in, 34; PET scans in, 35; ultrasound in, 35; X-rays in, 36

*Rain* (Sarsfield), 184*f*, 185

randomized, controlled clinical trials (RCTs), 12, 94; of Avastin, 60–63, 79*f*, 80–88; boundaries imposed in, 131; Cochrane Systematic Reviews of, 99; eligibility for participation in, 40; FDA hearings and, 69–71; meaningful endpoints in, 21, 61–64, 70*t*, 72, 75; publication of, 99; super-responders in, 66, 83–84. *See also* inferential statistics

recommendations for care. *See* synthesizing evidence

reference materials, 151–52, 157–63, 167–68, 213n15; as boundary objects, 161–62, 213n17; rhetorical infrastructure of, 162–63

*Reflected* (Sarsfield), 183*f*

relationality, 175

Rennie, D., 205n1

RevMan software, 97, 101, 106

rhetoric, 20–21, 56; definitions of, 76–77, 139; epistemological and ontological work of, 93, 139–40, 209n16

rhetorical work of biomedical practitioners, 2–4, 20–23, 171–72, 205n11, 208n7; in assessing evidence, 65–68, 76, 89–93, 169–70, 209n16; computational boundary work in, 139–40, 161–68, 170, 213nn17–20; dwelling with disease and, 175–85; enthymematic reasoning and, 171–72; ethic of care in, 167–68, 173–75; ethos of special warrants in, 92–93; as kairotic attunement, 23, 28, 52–59, 169; in managing risk, 165, 213n19; *phronesis* in, 21, 23, 25, 167, 177–82; as presence, 55–57; rhetorical attunement in, 171–85; in standards of care, 130–33; stasis theory and, 105, 127–30; in synthesizing evidence, 103–30, 170; Toulminian analysis of, 21, 24, 105, 115–27. *See also* evidential attunement

Rice, I., 139

Rickert, T.: on ambient attunement, 19, 138–39; on attunement, 14–15; on complexity, 205n2; on doing rhetoric, 20–21, 56, 76, 92, 169, 208n7; on dwelling, 54; on *kairos*, 56–57; on probabilistic methods, 76

Rieke, R. D., 126–27

risk, 3, 58, 135, 166

risk analyses, 208n10

risk-benefit ratio (RBR), 70*t*, 71

Robb, J., 17

Rogers, Everett, 210n1

Rotman, B., 209n14

Russell, J., 131

Sackett, David L., 98

Salzberg, S., 119

Sanger dideoxy sequencing, 204

Sarsfield, Tracey, 183–85

Sauer, B. A., 46, 58

Saunders, B. F., 45–46, 52

Schattner, Elaine, 124–26

scientific indeterminacy, 2

Scott, J. B., 56, 78, 213n17

"Screening for Breast Cancer with Mammography (Review)" (Gøtzsche and Jørgensen), 105, 108–12*t*; CSR outline for, 199–201; on methodological shortcomings, 113, 123–26; stasis theory and, 127–30; Toulminian analysis of, 122–26

"Screening for Lung Cancer (Review)" (Manser et al.), 105, 108–12*t*; CSR outline for, 201–3; stasis theory and, 127–30; Toulminian analysis of, 116–19

"Screening for Prostate Cancer (Review)" (Ilic et al.), 105, 108–12*t*; CSR outline for, 197–99; stasis theory and, 127–30; Toulminian analysis of, 119–22

Secor, M., 128, 133, 170

shadow work, 17–20, 25, 163–67

Simmons, W. M., 90

*Situational Analysis* (Clarke), 144, 146

situational mapping of genetic testing, 25, 144–61, 212n10; conceptual toolbox in, 146*f*, 147, 148*f*; definitions and examples in, 147–49, 150–51*t*; differing algorithms and computational codes in, 152–56, 212nn11–14; methodology of, 144–47; objects of study in, 148; overlapping discourse universes in, 158–61; polymorphic variations and, 156–58; reference materials databases and, 149–52, 157–63, 167–68, 213n15

Smith, D. L., 177–78

Smith, R., 205n1

SNP (single nucleotide polymorphism) genotyping, 151–53, 156, 212n11. *See also* genetic testing

Sophocles, 176

special warrants, 91–92

Spinuzzi, C., 143–44

Spruance, S. L., et al., 84

standards of care: algorithmic protocols and, 13–14; rhetorical nature of, standards of care (*continued*) 130–33; in tumor board conferences, 8, 44–45t, 45–46

Star, S. L., 17, 161–63

stasis theory, 64, 105, 126–30, 170

statistical analysis. *See* inferential statistics

statistical power, 85

statistical significance, 81, 86–89

Steinberg, D. L., 160

Strauss, A. L., 29–30, 69

suasive potential, 16–17, 20

super-responders, 66, 83–84

surrogate endpoints, 60, 62

survival rates, 62, 72, 79f, 80–83

synthesizing evidence, 2, 4, 21–24, 94–133, 167; Cochrane Systematic Review in, 24, 94–103; critiques of cut-making procedures in, 130–33; evidential attunement in, 131–33; labor of making evidential cuts in, 95–96, 105–6, 113–15, 118–30, 197–203; materiality of the corporeal body and, 126; as meta-analysis, 98; qualitative evidence in, 132–33; rhetorical analysis of, 103–30, 170; in standards of care, 130–33; stasis theory in, 105, 127–30; Toulminian analysis in, 24, 105, 115–16, 170

Syverson, M., 15

TallBear, Kim, 11, 143, 157, 166

*technai*, 176–77

"Thing, The" (Heidegger), 18

Toulminian analysis, 21, 24, 105, 115–27, 170; of extratextual features of CSRs, 115–16; on hitting on new ideas, 126–27; model of argumentation of, 105, 115–16; on probabilistic assessment, 76; of "Screening for Breast Cancer with Mammography" CSR, 122–26; of "Screening for Lung Cancer" CSR,

116–19; of "Screening for Prostate Cancer" CSR, 119–22; stasis theory and, 127–30

*tuche*, 176–77

tumor board conferences, 7–8, 205nn2–3; body data in, 7–8, 49–52; case deliberations in, 41–52; observational heuristics and mapping of, 29–30; process used in, 27–33; radiological-pathological references of, 31t; standards of care in, 8, 45–46; survival statistics in, 8; temporal periods of deliberation on images in, 32t

Tversky, A., 74–75, 76

23andMe, 140–42, 149; disclaimer of, 141, 163, 211n5; DNA profiling by, 151–53, 156, 212n11; financial backers of, 159; HaploScore algorithm of, 153–54

type I errors (α), 82

type II errors (β), 82

tyromancy, 9

ultrasound, 35

uncertainty, 1–2, 8, 58, 143

uncontrolled studies, 118–19

universes of discourses, 158–61

U.S. Supreme Court, 211n7

visualizing evidence, 2, 4, 21–23, 27–59, 206n3, 206nn6–7; in case deliberations, 41–52; evidencing (as practice) in, 54; kairotic attunement to, 23, 28, 52–59, 169; pathology imaging in, 33, 36–41; radiology imaging in, 33–36

Walker, Jeffrey, 78

Walker, K., 127

Walsh, L., 127

Watson, James, 136–37

Weinberg, R., 207n11

Weiser, M., 11

Welhausen, C. A., 208n8

Wells, H. G., 173

Winance, M., 180

Witte, Stephen P., 26–27, 46

Woolgar, S., 17, 134

*World on Paper* (Olson), 7

Wynn, J., 91–92

X-rays, 35, 36

Ziliak, S. T., 91